Histories of HIV/AIDS in Western Europe

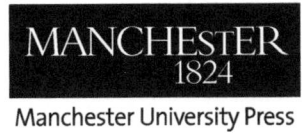

Manchester University Press

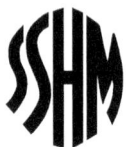

SOCIAL HISTORIES OF MEDICINE

Series editors: David Cantor, Elaine Leong and Keir Waddington

Social Histories of Medicine is concerned with all aspects of health, illness and medicine, from prehistory to the present, in every part of the world. The series covers the circumstances that promote health or illness, the ways in which people experience and explain such conditions, and what, practically, they do about them. Practitioners of all approaches to health and healing come within its scope, as do their ideas, beliefs, and practices, and the social, economic and cultural contexts in which they operate. Methodologically, the series welcomes relevant studies in social, economic, cultural, and intellectual history, as well as approaches derived from other disciplines in the arts, sciences, social sciences and humanities. The series is a collaboration between Manchester University Press and the Society for the Social History of Medicine.

Previously published

Migrant architects of the NHS   *Julian M. Simpson*

Mediterranean quarantines, 1750–1914   *Edited by John Chircop and Francisco Javier Martínez*

Sickness, medical welfare and the English poor, 1750–1834   *Steven King*

Medical societies and scientific culture in nineteenth-century Belgium   *Joris Vandendriessche*

Vaccinating Britain   *Gareth Millward*

Madness on trial   *James E. Moran*

Early Modern Ireland and the world of medicine   *Edited by John Cunningham*

Feeling the strain   *Jill Kirby*

Rhinoplasty and the nose in early modern British medicine and culture   *Emily Cock*

Communicating the history of medicine   *Edited by Solveig Jülich and Sven Widmalm*

Progress and pathology   *Edited by Melissa Dickson, Emilie Taylor-Brown and Sally Shuttleworth*

Balancing the self   *Edited by Mark Jackson and Martin D. Moore*

Global health and the new world order   *Edited by Jean-Paul Gaudillière, Claire Beaudevin, Christoph Gradmann, Anne M. Lovell and Laurent Pordié*

Accounting for health: Calculation, paperwork and medicine, 1500–2000   *Edited by Axel C. Hüntelmann and Oliver Falk*

Women's medicine   *Caroline Rusterholz*

Germs and governance: The past, present and future of hospital infection, prevention and control   *Edited by Anne Marie Rafferty, Marguerite Dupree and Fay Bound Alberti*

Leprosy and identity in the Middle Ages: From England to the Mediterranean   *Edited by Elma Brenner and François-Olivier Touati*

Patient voices in Britain, 1840–1948   *Edited by Anne Hanley and Jessica Meyer*

Medical histories of Belgium: New narratives on health, care and citizenship in the nineteenth and twentieth centuries   *Edited by Joris Vandendriessche and Benoît Majerus*

Histories of HIV/AIDS in Western Europe

New and regional perspectives

Edited by

Janet Weston and Hannah J. Elizabeth

MANCHESTER UNIVERSITY PRESS

Copyright © Manchester University Press 2022

While copyright in the volume as a whole is vested in Manchester University Press, copyright in individual chapters belongs to their respective authors.

Electronic versions of chapters 3, 4, 6, 7 and 8 have been made freely available under a Creative Commons (CC BY-NC-ND) licence, thanks to the support of the following: the Wellcome Trust (Chapter 3 under grant number 103341/Z/13/Z, Chapter 4 under grant number 222230/Z/20/Z and Chapter 6 under grant number 219747/Z/19/Z); Humanities in the European Research Area (Chapter 7 under grant HERA.15.093); and NWO, the Dutch Research Council (Chapter 8). This permits non-commercial use, distribution and reproduction provided the editor(s), chapter author(s) and Manchester University Press are fully cited and no modifications or adaptations are made. Details of the licence can be viewed at https://creativecommons.org/licenses/by-nc-nd/4.0/

Published by Manchester University Press
Oxford Road, Manchester M13 9PL

www.manchesteruniversitypress.co.uk

British Library Cataloguing-in-Publication Data
A catalogue record for this book is available from the British Library

ISBN 978 1 5261 5121 6 hardback

First published 2022

The publisher has no responsibility for the persistence or accuracy of URLs for any external or third-party internet websites referred to in this book, and does not guarantee that any content on such websites is, or will remain, accurate or appropriate.

Typeset by Newgen Publishing UK

Contents

List of figures	vii
List of tables	ix
List of contributors	x
Foreword – Virginia Berridge	xiv
Acknowledgements	xix
Abbreviations	xx
Introduction – Janet Weston and Hannah J. Elizabeth	1
1 Selling sex in the age of HIV/AIDS: activism, politics, and medicine in Norway, 1983–90 – Ketil Slagstad and Anne Kveim Lie	27
2 Drug criminalisation, the Catholic Church, and the 1988 founding of a Rome AIDS care centre – Brian DeGrazia	59
3 Responding to HIV/AIDS in European prisons, 1980s–2000s – Janet Weston	82
4 Nursing a plague: nurses' perspectives on their work during the United Kingdom HIV/AIDS crisis, 1981–96 – Tommy Dickinson, Nathan Appasamy, Lee P. Pritchard, and Laura Savidge	109
5 A phoney war? Health, education, and popular responses to HIV/AIDS in Wales, 1983–2003 – Daryl Leeworthy	139
6 Recovering mothers' experiences of HIV/AIDS health activism in Edinburgh, 1983–2000 – Hannah J. Elizabeth	164

7 The European HIV/AIDS Archive: building a queer counter-memory – Agata Dziuban, Eugen Januschke, Ulrike Klöppel, Todd Sekuler, and Justyna Struzik   192

8 Pandemics and national pride: collecting and curating the history of HIV/AIDS – Manon S. Parry   215

Index   236

Figures

1.1 'Jeg har aids', *Dagbladet*, 29 June 1985.
Reproduced with permission from *Dagbladet*   35
1.2 'Jeg er en levende dødsmaskin', *Dagbladet*,
6 August 1985. Reproduced with permission
from *Dagbladet*   36
1.3 'Kjøpte sex av aidshore', *VG*, 20 May 1988.
Reproduced with permission from Verdens Gang AS   38
1.4 'Du kan kjøpe deg AIDS-smitte', Norwegian Directorate of Health, 1987. Reproduced with permission from the Norwegian Directorate of Health, copyright ScanPartner/Anneks RRA6/Helsedirektoratet   47
1.5 'Du kan kjøpe deg AIDS-smitte', Norwegian Directorate of Health, 11 February 1987. Reproduced with permission from the Norwegian Directorate of Health, copyright ScanPartner/Anneks RRA6/Helsedirektoratet   48
2.1 'AIDS: Non si vede ma sta crescendo', Italian Health Ministry, 1990   70
2.2 'AIDS: Non si vede ma sta crescendo', Italian Health Ministry, 1990   71
4.1 Sean Pert and Darren, circa 1993/4. From the private collection of Sean Pert, reproduced with his kind permission   120
4.2 David (lying down) and Eric (sitting) at their home in Boston, 1986. Reproduced with permission by Sage Sohier, from her series 'At Home with Themselves: Same-Sex couples in 1980s America'   130

8.1 First panel of the exhibition *AIDS in Amsterdam, 1981–1996*, courtesy of exhibition designer Jasper van Goor and Amsterdam City Archives 226
8.2 Last panel of the exhibition *AIDS in Amsterdam, 1981–1996*, courtesy of exhibition designer Jasper van Goor and Amsterdam City Archives 227

Tables

5.1 HIV-positive results in Wales, 1984–94 141
5.2 HIV-positive individuals resident in Wales, 1997–2007 148

Contributors

Nathan Appasamy is a King's Undergraduate Research Fellow in the Florence Nightingale Faculty of Nursing, Midwifery and Palliative Care at King's College London.

Virginia Berridge is Professor of History and Health Policy at the London School of Hygiene & Tropical Medicine. She was co-director of the AIDS Social History Programme from 1988 to 1994, and later the director of the Centre for History in Public Health. She is the author of *AIDS in the UK: the making of policy, 1981–1994* (1996) and has published many other books and articles on public health and health policy, including *Demons: our changing attitudes to alcohol, tobacco and drugs* (2013) and *Public health: a very short introduction* (2016).

Brian DeGrazia is an independent scholar and translator. He holds a PhD in Italian Studies from New York university, where he wrote a dissertation about HIV/AIDS, the media, and biopolitical thought in Italy. In addition to his research on HIV/AIDS, Brian has published articles about academic labour and doctoral education in outlets such as Inside Higher Ed and the Los Angeles Review of Books.

Tommy Dickinson is a Reader in Nursing Education and Head of the Department of Mental Health Nursing in the Florence Nightingale Faculty of Nursing, Midwifery and Palliative Care at King's College London. In 2018, he was appointed as the Endowed Talbott Visiting Professor of Nursing at the University of Virginia

School of Nursing. Dr Dickinson is a Fellow of the American Academy of Nursing and a Fellow of the European Academy of Nursing Science.

Agata Dziuban is a sociologist, outreach worker, and Assistant Professor at the Institute of Sociology at the Jagiellonian University in Krakow. Her research projects focus on sex workers' self-organisation in Europe, the working conditions of migrant sex workers in Poland, and the making of HIV-related policies. Together with Todd Sekuler, she worked on European-level research within the 'Disentangling European HIV/AIDS policies: activism, citizenship and health' (EUROPACH) project.

Hannah J. Elizabeth is a historian of emotions and health working at the London School of Hygiene & Tropical Medicine on the Wellcome Trust-funded project 'What's Love Got To Do With It? Building and Maintaining HIV-Affected Families through Love, Care and Activism in Edinburgh, 1981–2016'.

Eugen Januschke studied mathematics and holds a doctoral degree in philosophy. He is an activist in the field of AIDS remembrance. His current research, which is based out of the Institute for European Ethnology at Humboldt-Universität zu Berlin, focuses on the history of AIDS activism in Germany.

Ulrike Klöppel holds a doctoral degree in sociology. Her research focuses on the medicalisation of intersex and gender transition in the German Democratic Republic, gender and queer history, and the history of psychiatry. Her ongoing research project at the Humboldt-Universität zu Berlin is about the history of AIDS activism in Germany.

Daryl Leeworthy is the Rhys Davies Trust Research Fellow at Swansea University and the author of several books on modern Britain, including *A little gay history of Wales* (2019) and *Labour country: political radicalism and social democracy in South Wales, 1831–1985* (2018), as well as numerous articles and chapters on the social, political, and queer history of modern Britain.

Anne Kveim Lie is a physician and historian, working as an Associate Professor in Medical History at the Department of Community Medicine and Global Health at the University of Oslo. She is particularly interested in how diseases, medical practices, and medical technology come into being. Among her research interests are the history of (bio)medicalisation, the history of reproduction, and the history of infectious diseases including syphilis and antibiotic resistance.

Manon S. Parry is Professor of Medical History at the Free University Amsterdam and Senior Lecturer in American Studies and Public History at the University of Amsterdam. She was previously curator in the History of Medicine Division of the National Library of Medicine, Maryland. She is co-editor of *Women physicians and the cultures of medicine* (Johns Hopkins University Press, 2008), winner of the Archivists and Librarians in the History of the Health Sciences Publication Award for Best Print Publication in 2012, and author of *Broadcasting birth control: family planning and mass media* (2013). Her current research project is 'Human curiosities: expanding the social relevance of medical museums'.

Lee P. Pritchard is an English teacher at Woodford County High School for Girls in London.

Laura Savidge is a Nursing student in the Florence Nightingale Faculty of Nursing, Midwifery and Palliative Care at King's College London.

Todd Sekuler holds a master's in Public Health and a doctoral degree in European Ethnology. Together with Agata Dziuban, he has been conducting research on HIV/AIDS policy worlds at the European level as part of the transnational research project 'Disentangling European HIV/AIDS policies: activism, citizenship and health' (EUROPACH).

Ketil Slagstad is a physician and former Editor of the *Journal of the Norwegian Medical Association*. His research interests include the history of social medicine, the history of biomedicalisation, and the history of HIV/AIDS. He is undertaking a PhD in the history of science and medicine, addressing the emergence of transgender medicine in Scandinavia in the second half of the 20th century.

Justyna Struzik received her PhD in Sociology from the Institute of Sociology at Jagiellonian University in Kracow with the thesis 'Queer movements in Poland'. Between 2016 and 2019 she was a postdoctoral researcher on the project 'Disentangling European HIV/AIDS policies: activism, citizenship and health' (EUROPACH). She is the co-author of *Różnym głosem. Rodziny z wyboru w Polsce (In different voices: families of choice in Poland*, 2017) with Joanna Mizielińska and Agnieszka Król, and the author of *Solidarność queerowa. Mobilizacja, ramy i działania ruchów queerowych w Polsce (Queer solidarity: mobilisation, frames and actions of queer movements in Poland*, 2019).

Janet Weston is an Assistant Professor at the London School of Hygiene & Tropical Medicine. Her research, funded by the Wellcome Trust, addresses histories of health, medicine, and law, with a particular focus on mental illness, prisons, crime, ethics, and sexuality. She is the author of *Medicine, sexual crime, and the penal system in England, 1919–1960s* (2018).

Foreword

Virginia Berridge

History has played a significant role in the understanding of and response to HIV/AIDS. In the early days, back in the mid-1980s, it was history *and* AIDS. How could history feed into our understanding of this looming epidemic in the present? How could we use responses to past epidemics or to sexually transmitted disease to help provide blueprints for the present to emulate or to avoid?

Then came the idea that the advent of HIV/AIDS was a memorable historical event in its own right. History of AIDS replaced history and AIDS. The AIDS Social History Programme (ASHP) at the London School of Hygiene & Tropical Medicine (LSHTM), of which I was co-director, began in the late 1980s. Funded by the Nuffield Trust (then the Nuffield Provincial Hospitals Trust), it was set up to study 'history in the making' – to study over a five-year period of funding (lavish in those days) events which had yet to happen when the research programme began. That was an unusual situation for an historian to find herself in. Even now, it is uncommon for people to consider the study of such events as 'history'. At the time, phrases such as 'journalist history' or 'the first draft of history' were used to denote the difficult terrain our programme was traversing. But of course, we also had the opportunity, situated in a leading UK school of public health, to have a ringside seat as events unfolded, with access to key players in policy and research terms. And historical analysis and awareness is indeed possible, even if one is studying the events of the day before.

At that time, too, there was an archival consciousness. People were aware that they were living through life-changing events and that memories might soon fade. What would be kept to ensure that future generations knew what had happened, what people had lived through? The ASHP had a consultant archivist, Janet Foster, who early on produced a brief pamphlet (before the days of the internet) listing relevant organisations and what they had kept, but also with an advisory function, addressing what to focus on keeping and what was less central.[1]

But then came change. As Janet Weston and Hannah J. Elizabeth comment in their Introduction, interest in HIV/AIDS died away as the predicted epidemic in Western countries did not materialise, as treatments came on-line, and as the imagery of chronic disease replaced that of epidemic catastrophe. When my book on AIDS policy-making was published in 1996, it was greeted with sharp-eyed cynicism in one interview with a leading health journalist. Hadn't it all been a gigantic fuss about nothing, he asked, a complete waste of money? Gay men's propaganda had diverted government away from the real issues. Why had my book not taken that line? This was an unpromising time to launch a book which did not replicate the then-received opinion but, rather, looked at how the British government had responded in all its complexity to a major health crisis, at how the apparent Thatcherite revolution in government had encompassed a liberal policy response strangely at odds with its public persona.[2] That type of history was certainly off the agenda in the mid-1990s.

Now, as our editors have reminded us and the contents of this book demonstrate, there is a revival of historical interest. Years have passed and a historical approach is more acceptable. The contents of the book show that this is the case; there is also a growth in interest in television and radio series focused on HIV/AIDS. That historical interest still has a particular focus, which is primarily on gay men and their experience of the epidemic. Drug users and haemophiliacs are of relatively little interest in that context; they remain 'hidden from history'. A television researcher who approached the LSHTM archive and myself for access to the interviews which I had done as part of the ASHP told me she was not interested in those groups. The idea of 'legitimation through disaster', the process which took place for gay men through HIV/AIDS, had no such enduring impact for them. This is in part because, in their case, the epidemic has not ended, as demonstrated by the Infected Blood Inquiry in the UK and its evidence and the ongoing debates round harm reduction tactics in Scotland. So it is good to see drug users and prison inmates feature in this book. What is remembered and what is not, as our editors comment, is a partial matter.

This book highlights the regional and the local in its study of HIV/AIDS. This was always a feature of the response, right from the start. My interviews from the 1980s and 1990s have contemporaneous material on the local response in Exeter, in Cardiff, in Brighton, and in Edinburgh. The following is a flavour of the Cardiff recollection.

> We wanted to establish a helpline because we felt that if we didn't do it, as members of Friend, then some other organisation may take it on-board and they may not be as sort of understanding and sympathetic to the issue as we felt we were with Friend. I remember we contacted Powys Health Authority who told us that it wasn't a problem because gay homosexuals didn't exist in Powys. We were up against that attitude and that is with the people, 'it is not a problem, it is not going to happen here, therefore go away, we cannot fund you'. Then on the last day of the financial year, it was 31 March 1986, I had a phone call from Bob Goosy, the Health Promotion Officer, who said 'get down here quick, I've got two grand left, get it into Friend's account today or you lose it'. So he had managed to get two thousand pounds for us, which we put in Cardiff Friend's account for the purpose of starting Cardiff AIDS Helpline. You see the Health Authority was saying 'you start the Helpline and then we will see how it goes and then we will fund you'. And we were saying 'no we won't establish the Helpline until you fund us', because we felt that once we established the group, because we were funding Cardiff Friends out of our own pockets. There were about fifteen members of Friend and we were giving five pounds a month towards the running costs of the group, so we were always in dire financial hardship. We were using a room in this hospital, one room that they gave us rent-free.[3]

Such actions linked into activism, and into national but also international networks, as the editors remind us. One aspect of the early response to HIV/AIDS was indeed this internationalism. In part this was shown through the traditional international organisations such as the World Health Organization (WHO) and later the Joint United Nations Programme on HIV/AIDS (UNAIDS), disseminating an international ethic of non-discrimination and human rights. But there were also international activist networks which pre-dated HIV/AIDS, as in the case of drug users, which is emphasised in this collection. There was also a strong interest early on in the comparative study of policy towards HIV/AIDS. A raft of books appeared in the early 1990s, contrasting the policy response in different countries, a focus which was less obvious as time went on.[4] Overall, in fact, a shift can be discerned away from policy and towards the cultural aspects of HIV/AIDS, which were also significant in the early days.[5] The differences between countries are one key feature of this book, with an emphasis on countries in Western Europe. This reflects pre-Brexit academic study in the UK, when European networks were in place and comparisons were possible. The focus had perhaps moved elsewhere after the 1990s, with HIV/AIDS in African countries and in Southeast Asia receiving more academic attention. The Western European perspective will now be more difficult to maintain, as the focus of research and funding moves.

This book's gestation has weathered the advent of Covid-19 and the impact that it has had on society. It is too early to say what the long-term cultural impact of Covid will be, but there are some interesting reflections and comparisons with the long-term response to HIV/AIDS. Quarantine and punitive social restrictions are so very different from the emphasis on human rights and a non-punitive response which marked many official responses to HIV/AIDS. Covid has been a more traditional public health issue, with these very long-standing methods of coercive control centre stage. Yet, other issues which could not be spoken of in the 1980s have been openly discussed in relation to Covid. Race was deliberately downplayed in official public health work in the case of HIV/AIDS in the UK, for fear of a social backlash. Thirty or more years on, racial disparities in infection have been explicitly acknowledged for Covid. The local has been important for both, although in the 1980s it was local activism around HIV/AIDS which was important, whereas in 2020 it was local epidemiology and local public health teams which figured more prominently. Archives and the nature of remembrance have come to the fore, with Covid initiatives stimulated by the memory of what had been done for HIV/AIDS. Differences between countries and their policies have been much discussed, possibly to a greater degree at a global level than they were for HIV/AIDS. But activism on the scale witnessed for HIV/AIDS has been almost completely lacking for Covid. Only the 'anti-vaxxers' take up the banner of opposition to restrictions on individual liberty, but from a different perspective to those who defended human rights in relation to HIV/AIDS.

The editors and authors of this book are to be congratulated for their contribution to 'second-wave' histories of HIV/AIDS.

Notes

1 Janet Foster, *AIDS archives in the UK* (London: AIDS Social History Programme, 1990).
2 Virginia Berridge, *AIDS in the UK: the making of policy, 1981–1994* (Oxford: Oxford University Press, 1996).
3 Interview with member of Cardiff AIDS helpline by Janet Foster, 21 February 1991.
4 Barbara A. Miztal and David Moss (eds), *Action on AIDS: national policies in comparative perspective* (New York: Greenwood Press, 1990); Mildred Blaxter, *AIDS: worldwide policies and problems* (London: Office of Health Economics, 1990); David L. Kirp and Ronald Bayer, *AIDS in the industrialised democracies: passions, politics, and policies* (New Brunswick, NJ: Rutgers University Press, 1992).
5 Peter Aggleton and Hilary Homans (eds), *Social aspects of AIDS* (London: The Falmer Press, 1988).

Acknowledgements

Funding from the Wellcome Trust, the Humanities in the European Research Area (HERA) network, and NWO, the Dutch Research Council, means that five of the chapters in this collection are freely available under a Creative Commons (CC BY-NC-ND) licence; we are pleased to acknowledge this financial support.

We are very grateful to all those who participated in the symposium that inspired this collection, held at Birkbeck, University of London, in July 2018 and supported by funding from the Society for the Social History of Medicine and the Birkbeck Institute for the Humanities. We would also like to acknowledge the work of all those who contributed to the broader Festival of AIDS Cultures and Histories taking place across London at the same time, under the aegis of the Raphael Samuel History Centre; this festival provided an inspiring context in which to reassess histories of HIV/AIDS. In particular, our thanks go to Matt Cook for initiating the festival and symposium and encouraging us in the production of this collection, and to Katy Pettit for her unfailing good humour and flawless administrative skills. Special thanks are due to all of the contributors to this collection for their patience and commitment in the face of a new pandemic, which caused countless delays and difficulties. Your enthusiasm and dedication to the project have made the potentially tough business of lockdown editing a true pleasure.

Abbreviations

AIDS	acquired immune deficiency syndrome
Anlaids	L'Associazione nazionale per la lotta contro l'Aids
ASHP	AIDS Social History Programme
CDC	Centers for Disease Control and Prevention
DHSS	Department of Health and Social Security
EATG	European AIDS Treatment Group
ECS	European Collaborative Study
EHAA	European HIV/AIDS Archive
HIV	human immunodeficiency viruses
HLTV-III	human T-lymphotropic virus type III
IAS	International AIDS Society
IV	intravenous
GDR	German Democratic Republic
LGBT	lesbian, gay, bisexual, trans*
LHB	Lothian Health Board
LSHTM	London School of Hygiene & Tropical Medicine
MSM	men who have sex with men
MuCEM	Museum of European and Mediterranean Civilizations
PARC	Paediatric AIDS Resource Centre
PrEP	pre-exposure prophylaxis
PWHA	people living with HIV/AIDS
RCN	Royal College of Nursing
RN	registered nurse
THT	Terrence Higgins Trust
UK	United Kingdom
UNAIDS	Joint United Nations Programme on HIV/AIDS
USA	United States of America
WHO	World Health Organization

Introduction

Janet Weston and Hannah J. Elizabeth

As we write, the fortieth anniversary of the first confirmed cases of what we now call acquired immune deficiency syndrome (AIDS) is rapidly approaching. This marks four decades of pandemic AIDS and human immunodeficiency virus (HIV), resulting in an estimated global death toll of 32 million.[1] There have now been decades of biomedical research and innovation tackling the virus and its effects, but also decades of activism and campaigning, of creativity and cultural production, of learning and sharing knowledge. At regional, national, and global levels, countless laws, policies, and practices which touch on every aspect of life from immigration to employment to the family have come under scrutiny in the wake of the crisis and, in some cases, have undergone radical change. Most recently, questions of remembering and forgetting have come to the fore through memorials, exhibitions, and newly established archives.[2] This milestone therefore also marks nearly forty years of arts, humanities, and social science work that responds to HIV and AIDS.

From its earliest days, the political, cultural, and social aspects of HIV/AIDS were recognised, and historical analysis played a central role.[3] A revival of historical interest in the epidemic is now taking place, as the distance of decades provides new perspectives, new sources, new anxieties about the ephemera and oral histories that vanish with every passing day, and a new generation of researchers looking with fresh eyes at a crisis older than they are. As we enter the 2020s, salutary reminders of the policies, problems, and prejudices summoned forth by new infectious diseases are abundant and may continue to prompt attention to the crises of the past.

It is therefore a suitable moment to offer a collection that showcases some of this new historical work on HIV/AIDS. Our aim is to introduce aspects of much less well-known histories and legacies, whether that be in terms of place or people involved. Most of Western Europe, our geographic focus, encountered HIV/AIDS at around the same time and responded in broadly similar terms, but these similarities have obscured significant differences between regions and nations. The nature of, and reaction to, the emergence and spread of HIV/AIDS varied significantly according to place, as did the experiences of those affected by it both personally and professionally.

Although this book does not by any means offer a comprehensive view of HIV/AIDS across Western Europe, it begins to introduce histories from parts of this region where the events and policies of the epidemic are less familiar: Edinburgh, Wales, Rome, Norway, the Netherlands, Ireland, and Switzerland. It also draws attention to the experiences and activities of actors who feature much less prominently in existing histories. Although the epidemic disproportionately affected men who had sex with men (MSM), others were (and are) seriously affected, whether because of their perceived or actual risk of infection and transmission or their involvement in forms of care and activism. In this collection we highlight some examples of these lesser-known, but no less significant, histories with chapters that focus on sex workers, drug users, women, nurses, and those living and working in prisons. Finally, and relatedly, this book begins to probe the question of how HIV/AIDS in decades past is, or should be, remembered. As well as introducing new sources, archives, and disciplinary perspectives that offer ways of enriching future histories, these chapters also point towards the gaps that remain.

In this introductory chapter, we review some of the key moments in the last four decades of HIV/AIDS in Western Europe and the contours of existing histories of HIV/AIDS in the United Kingdom (UK) and United States of America (USA). We then unpack the idea of the 'AIDS capital' as a culturally constructed myth, deploying it as a starting point from which to expand on the insights and themes offered in this collection. As well as highlighting the importance of regional specificity, the collection explores different forms of activism, scrutinises less familiar strands of HIV/AIDS policy and research, and asks how (or whose) histories of HIV/AIDS are preserved and remembered. Questions of activism, policy, and commemoration have long been central to the stories told about this pandemic; we hope that this collection reintroduces them from new perspectives as topics worthy of close historical scrutiny.

A history of HIV/AIDS

The outline of the emergence and impact of HIV/AIDS is fairly well known. Initial newspaper and clinical reports appeared in the USA in mid-1981 noting clusters of unusual cancers, infections, and other symptoms among MSM and injecting drug users. Haemophiliacs were soon reported to be another group affected by these mystery ailments, as were Haitians.[4] Although initially denoted by various different terms and acronyms as researchers and clinicians struggled to get to grips with this new disease, the designation 'AIDS' was first introduced in 1982. The virus that was eventually named 'HIV' was identified by researchers in the USA and France the following year, and by 1985 a test for HIV had been developed and was being put to use across Western Europe. By this time, governmental responses remained limited, but charities and informal support groups led by people affected by HIV and AIDS had sprung up around the region. These early community responses frequently led the way in terms of delivering services and campaigns. With HIV testing providing insight into prevalence, and with confirmation that this was a blood-borne virus that anybody could acquire, much of the region saw a dramatic uptick in mainstream media attention in the mid-1980s. This attention often conveyed and evoked a sense of panic, fear, and disgust.

By the end of 1988, France had reported the highest number of persons with AIDS of all European nations gathering comparable data, at 3,073.[5] Data from Italy and Spain also indicated that those countries were severely affected, as were the UK and the Federal Republic of Germany. Governments began to take action, with state-funded public health campaigns launched in many countries. These campaigns often attempted to reach as wide an audience as possible through, for example, prime-time television broadcasts or billboard advertising. This higher profile was marked by the inauguration of World AIDS Day in 1988, organised by the World Health Organization (WHO)'s Global Programme on AIDS in order to raise awareness. This was also a time of emergent criminalisation, with some of the first cases in which individuals were prosecuted for transmitting HIV taking place in Germany, the Netherlands, and Switzerland.[6]

Campaigning, lobbying, national and local prevention efforts, and research all continued into the 1990s, but the fever pitch of the late 1980s had dissipated somewhat. By the late 1990s, treatments had improved dramatically with the arrival of highly active antiretroviral therapies (known as HAART) and HIV was on the road to becoming a manageable chronic condition for those with access to such drugs. The overarching story of the response to HIV/AIDS in Western Europe during these two decades has been characterised by the WHO as one of relative success, but between 1985 and 1991 the numbers of diagnoses and deaths were still vast: 112,000 HIV diagnoses, 76,000 individuals diagnosed with AIDS, and 39,000 deaths.[7] And, although fatalities declined dramatically from the mid-1990s, rates of HIV infection then began to rise again across much of the region as HIV/AIDS slipped from the headlines.[8] More recently, recommendations from the European Medicines Agency in 2016 for the use of certain drugs as pre-exposure prophylaxis (commonly known as PrEP) to reduce the risks of infection have opened the door to a new era of prevention, albeit one whose potential has not yet been fully realised. Rates of HIV infection in Western Europe declined between 2010 and 2020 and are rarely now a matter for headlines, but HIV/AIDS continues to have a disproportionate impact upon the most marginalised and regional variation remains stark.[9]

This snapshot of mounting crisis during the 1980s followed by a gradual and uneven tapering off as biomedical solutions took effect is largely drawn from the mainstream historical narratives of the epidemic as it played out in the UK and the USA. Its timeline focuses on technical innovations, with a sideline in changing attitudes and rates of death or infection. It depicts a situation that is now mostly under control. As the chapters here suggest, this much-simplified portrait is not entirely wrong when we start paying closer attention to regional and national specificities within Western Europe. Many of these key moments have resonance beyond borders, and developments in biomedical knowledge inevitably contributed to the overarching trajectory of the epidemic. Panic and fear were plentiful, and voluntary activities were often essential.

Yet this collection also shows that this is not the whole story. Progress or success is not always easy to discern. Support and action emerged from sometimes surprising quarters, while activism was not always immediately effective. Health authorities, governments, and other service providers were not uniformly recalcitrant and then panic-stricken; events were at times deeply entwined with national self-image, institutional structures, individual interventions, and politics at every level. Biomedical successes in combatting the virus reached different communities and regions at different times, and media responses, just like policy decisions, were inflected with local concerns, resulting in a plurality of trajectories and timelines. Memories and historical narratives are themselves diverse, fluctuating, and inevitably incomplete, reflecting experiences in the present and hopes for the future as well as changing understandings of the past. Historical work addressing regions, nations, and communities within Western Europe that are not covered here, including Germany, the Iberian peninsula, Northern Ireland, France, and rural areas across the region, along with migrants, children, faith communities, and people affected by haemophilia, will no doubt have many more lessons to share about this irregular landscape.

British and American histories have dominated English-language scholarship, at least until recent times. Historically informed analyses of HIV/AIDS appeared in the UK and USA as early as the mid-1980s, generated by sociologists, cultural and political theorists, and activists, as well as historians. Best-selling narratives of the epidemic such as activist-journalist Randy Shilts' *And the band played on*, published in 1987, were joined by rich academic work on the politics of HIV/AIDS, policy responses, and the ever-multiplying cultural representations of HIV/AIDS in film, television, art, music, and literature.[10] Anglo-American histories of medicine and sexuality hastily brought themselves up to date by incorporating HIV/AIDS, often framing it as the latest episode in a long story of stigmatisation hindering socio-medical responses to venereal disease, or medico-moral discourses dominating ideas of sexuality.[11] Feminists recognised yet another iteration of sexism at play in the politics of HIV/AIDS and the narratives which dominated scientific research, public health responses, and popular press coverage alike.[12] In relation to policy, the 'lessons of history' were called upon to influence official responses, pointing out the failure of punitive and stigmatising reactions to infectious disease in the past.[13] Soon thereafter, greater historical scrutiny of the emergent medical, political, and cultural responses to HIV/AIDS began to appear.[14]

In these early iterations, clinical, policy, and public responses were often situated in the context of long-standing moralising around sexuality and illness, not only within medicine but also public policy and the media. This reflected the early framing of HIV/AIDS as first and foremost a sexually transmitted infection and was interpreted by historians as part of a backlash against the liberatory advances of the 1960s and 1970s. Policy responses (or lack thereof) in the UK and USA were also interpreted in light of the rise of the new right, as reflected in the electoral victories of Ronald Reagan and Margaret Thatcher. But alongside this critique of government inaction and widespread stigmatisation were emergent accounts of HIV/AIDS as transformative. In this telling, HIV/AIDS marked the arrival of new forms of community support and mobilisation, new levels of acceptance of patient expertise, burgeoning attention to the interplay of health and human rights, and the revitalisation of gay activism.[15] Others explored the loosening of tongues in the public sphere around taboo subjects such as sex, drugs, and sexuality, suggesting that the necessity of talking plainly about HIV transmission allowed such topics to be confronted more openly.[16]

As HIV/AIDS gradually changed in the mainstream public imagination, fading from sudden and horrifying 'plague' to familiar fact of modern life, its histories changed too. They began to consider in more depth the extent to which HIV/AIDS had brought about medical and social change, and the forces that had shaped policy decisions, including the uses of history. They also identified distinct phases within the years of the pandemic, from a period of mounting fear and community action in the first half of the 1980s to a peak of panic around 1985, followed by government intervention, cultural mainstreaming, and the increasing professionalisation of services, campaigns, and expertise surrounding HIV/AIDS as well.[17] Such work also addressed issues and populations that slotted less easily into histories of HIV/AIDS that focused on sexuality, including its effects on drug policy and drug users, and women.

No sooner had this wider historical lens begun to appear than the profile of HIV/AIDS lessened in the UK and USA, as the fears and controversies it had once generated began to fade. Fatalities continued, of course, but as HIV became a manageable chronic condition for many in Western Europe and infection rates seemed to be under control, its profile declined. The waning of the sense of crisis, the fact that events and epidemiology seemed to have stabilised, and perhaps also an element of exhaustion after so much anxious scrutiny all prompted a quieter period for scholarship on the historical, cultural, and political context of HIV/AIDS. Cultural representations and reflections also largely disappeared for over a decade, generating that which writer and artist Theodore (ted) Kerr has dubbed a 'Second Silence' surrounding HIV/AIDS.[18]

The thirtieth anniversary of the beginnings of the HIV/AIDS crisis in the UK and USA saw a resurgence of popular attention to its history, with numerous memoirs, biographies, film and television treatments, documentaries, and exhibitions in the early 2010s.[19] A generation born into an era in which HIV/AIDS was simply a muted part of the landscape was coming of age, and there was a clear desire to ensure that the turmoil and suffering of the 1980s and early 1990s were not forgotten. New scholarly works began to emerge as well, albeit more slowly, as the 1980s and 1990s became the object of more general historical attention and reassessment.[20]

Some of this work has begun to challenge existing narratives of the early years of the crisis. Historian Richard A. McKay has used the popular and problematic narrative of an 'AIDS patient zero' to great effect to revisit early research and representations of HIV/AIDS in North America, and a roundtable discussion on 'HIV/AIDS and US history' in the *Journal of American History* in 2016 called for a revitalised history that would avoid past tendencies to focus on wealthy, white, gay men.[21] Importantly, histories with a national and archival focus beyond the UK or USA have also been published or translated, broadening the horizons of English-language scholarship beyond the English-speaking world.[22]

These recent works point towards some of the themes that we develop in this collection. What can we learn about HIV/AIDS by paying attention to different regional or national perspectives? What were the experiences of those whose encounters with HIV/AIDS are less well documented, and what forms of activism may have been forgotten? What new archives and resources are now available, and what has been or should be retained, archived, collected, and exhibited? Many of the chapters in this collection use archival methodologies, drawing on a variety of printed sources including the popular press, governmental archives and publications, and public health literature to analyse the past. But chapters also draw and reflect on newly assembled archives, recent exhibitions, oral histories, and the ephemeral material traces of HIV/AIDS, from telephone logs to children's workbooks. In keeping with the diverse disciplinary backgrounds of the contributors, this collection contains contrasting ideas about framing and interpreting these sources. With these materials and ideas at our disposal, how might we re-tell the histories of the epidemic?

Reframing the 'AIDS capital', reviving regional and marginalised perspectives

Histories of HIV/AIDS have often adopted a national perspective, but in the last decades of the twentieth century the media told a powerful story in which regional specificity and particular deviant populations were central to the story of the epidemic. In the British press, certain cities were depicted as paradigmatic of the issues surrounding HIV/AIDS, albeit different cities at different times. From the early days of the crisis, these urban centres formed the set dressing for many of the tawdry HIV/AIDS dramas recounted by a press revelling in the power of fear and prejudice to sell newspapers. The label 'AIDS capital' was stamped on Edinburgh, New York, San Francisco, Berne, Zurich, Amsterdam, and Kinshasa, to name but a few. This branding evoked ideas of urban decay and the dangers of modern life; an 'AIDS capital' was a sign of the times, providing evidence of the inevitable consequences of metropolitan excess, or proof that liberal politics and permissiveness would lead to ruin. It was a way to rebuke cities and their residents for their perceived failings, while providing reassurance for places and people that seemed to have little in common with any of the 'AIDS capitals' of the world and their denizens. Importantly, it pinned HIV/AIDS in place. The idea of an 'AIDS capital' made the problem geographically limited, constrained within city limits and often safely located among people and places 'elsewhere'.

Within this framing, HIV/AIDS became a symptom of the negative consequences of permissiveness, often appearing in the media to add colour to broader criticism. For example, in a scathing review of 'Sgt Pepper: it was twenty years ago today', a 1960s retrospective aired on UK television in 1987, journalist Mary Kenny offered the following conclusion: 'Perhaps it is too soon for an intelligent analytical programme on the consequences of the 1960s, beginning with Amsterdam in the days of hippy happenings, today a drug-ridden AIDS-infected capital of crime, anarchy and vice.'[23] Here, Amsterdam represented the worst of the modern era: a place where the recent excesses of liberalism and tolerance, with which the 1960s were associated, had led swiftly to disorder and disease. Similarly, in a *Sunday Times* book profile with no evident connection to the HIV/AIDS crisis, the mantle of 'AIDS capital' was presented as the tragic but inevitable outcome of the earlier counter-cultural movements and lifestyles that had dominated particular cities. Readers were told that San Francisco, once 'the capital of hippiedom[,] is now the capital of Aids. Ah well, it was good while it lasted.'[24] Such articles drew on earlier moral panics about hippies as counter-cultural figures, fixing them geographically to present a direct connection between counter-cultural movements and HIV/AIDS.[25] They also implied that HIV/AIDS was not something that could affect anyone but, rather, was associated only with particular kinds of people whose lives were far from the mainstream.

Similarly, the 'AIDS capital' label was deployed in articles discussing thriving art scenes, cementing a connection between cultural innovation, success, and disease. Edinburgh's Fringe Festival was rarely mentioned in the late 1980s without the tempering title, and San Francisco frequently received similar treatment.[26] The arts, with their reputation for greater tolerance for gender, sexual, social, and political non-conformity, were by implication another specific context – often urban – in which the dissolute and diseased might take root.

This narrative of urban permissiveness and transgressive lifestyles creating the conditions for a localised HIV/AIDS crisis also allowed the 'AIDS capital' label to function as a warning. In a British newspaper article from 1989 which attempted to instil fear in its readers by using racist stereotypes alongside melodramatic descriptions of urban decay, New York's status as the 'AIDS capital of the world' was offered up as a dire warning of future calamity. New York had once been a cultural capital of the world, but now the only culture which New York is offering to the world is one of violence, of the degradation of drugs, of a yawning division between the revoltingly rich and the hopelessly poor – a culture, in short, of headlong moral decay which none of us wants to emulate. The city of dreams has now become the city of nightmares ... And since New York has so often been a foretaste of all our tomorrows, it is a torment whose bitter cup we shall soon drink to the dregs unless we are both vigilant and lucky.[27]

Thus the media suggested that it was not only HIV/AIDS that would spread between cities, but also a kind of social, moral collapse. Similarities between San Francisco or New York and assorted European cities were darkly invoked.

At the same time, the idea of an 'AIDS capital' could secure the epidemic and the worst of its dangers elsewhere, in cities and among people depicted as fundamentally different. Kinshasa, branded the 'Aids capital of Africa' by *The Times* in 1986, was presented as home to dangerous medical procedures and rampant sexual promiscuity, both of which were said to have caused exceptionally high rates of HIV infection. Even the 'maternal instincts' of the 'African women' in this city were flawed, prompting them to 'choose injections rather than pills for their sick babies', with terrible consequences. The sombre warning emanating from this AIDS capital was that richer nations should be sure to give something back, as they reaped the benefits of HIV/AIDS research conducted in this most dangerous of cities.[28] Notably, those richer nations were not themselves at risk of a similar fate.

The concept of the 'AIDS capital' also gave a regional colour to reportage. Reporters used the presence of HIV/AIDS as shorthand for a city's seedy underbelly while they built on regional stereotypes, or, even more dramatically, implied that HIV/AIDS was poised to transform any positive stereotypes for good. 'Switzerland, better known as the country of cuckoo clocks, secret bank accounts and trains that run on time', began a *Sunday Times* article from 1987, 'has one of the highest heroin addiction rates in Europe – and it has now become the Aids capital of Europe, too'. Taking a similar track, the *Daily Mail* reported in 1992 that Zurich's so-called 'Needle Park'

> has finally shattered the chocolate-box image of an Alpine paradise: the serpent of AIDS and drug-addiction has now entered Eden. ...

Introduction   11

[W]hen young people from all over Europe and North Africa think of Switzerland they don't think of edelweiss – they think of heroin. Instead of cuckoo clocks they think of cocaine and crack.[29]

Such reports revelled in the contrast between Switzerland's staid international reputation and the spectre of addiction and HIV/AIDS. The message was clear. Even sensible Switzerland could be swept up in this maelstrom of urban decay and liberal drug policies, with potentially disastrous effects for its international standing.

In a similar vein, Edinburgh was often depicted as duplicitous because of its wealth and beauty alongside its high rates of HIV. Edinburgh's grandeur was contrasted dramatically with the dire straits in which the city's drug users found themselves. One particularly lurid and unsympathetic description of this contrasting urban experience was offered by the *Daily Mail* in 1986.

George and Neil don't care. … they share no pride in Edinburgh's grandeur and tradition. George and Neil are heroin addicts. They are also AIDS carriers. Teenagers like them with dirty heroin needles, smacked out afternoons and prospects of the withering, life-sucking progress of the most feared disease on earth are becoming the main topic of conversation in this elegant city.[30]

Edinburgh's beautiful buildings were also contrasted with 'the rotting concrete and glass council estates that circle the city', where 'the virus incubates and spreads through the dirty needles of drug-addict tenants'. These tenants were then described with gothic sensationalism as 'addicts hunched in dark corners and abandoned flats, the scabs on their arms and ankles glowing raw red from their pale skin'.[31] In this presentation, HIV/AIDS threatened to transform the city, as the 'rot' emanating from distinctly modern concrete-and-glass council estates encircled the stylish old city centre. The residents of these estates, 'addicts' and 'AIDS carriers', were placed at arm's length, disconnected from the city's past and excluded from its present-day conversations – alarming, but apart.

The use of the 'AIDS capital' label in the British media signalled a desire to pin HIV/AIDS down to specific places and types of person, from mothers in Kinshasa to drug addicts in Swiss parks. These media depictions are not only powerfully indicative of some of the anxieties that swirled around HIV/AIDS in the 1980s and early 1990s in the UK, but also raise questions about a wider array of places and people than are usually associated with the history of HIV/AIDS. Did the epidemic in fact have a significant impact on mothers, or drug users? Were experiences in Edinburgh unusual, sharing more with Zurich than Glasgow or London? The connections and conclusions drawn by the press may have been ill-informed and their characterisations lazy, but rates of HIV/AIDS, activist and policy responses, and the experiences of those affected certainly did vary from place to place. The troublesome concept of an 'AIDS capital', brought into being when too much acceptance of difference supposedly led to moral and even structural collapse, calls attention to the possibility of regional variation and serves as a reminder of the many different marginalised groups that were so often implicated. What happened in regions like Wales or Norway that consistently evaded any 'AIDS capital' branding? How did people in 'AIDS capitals' like Amsterdam see their national response to HIV/AIDS? What services were provided to those in the media spotlight, including sex workers, heroin users, young people, and the 'hopelessly poor'? Do our histories and memories threaten to exclude some places or people, or flatten the complexities and ambiguities of HIV/AIDS activism, policy, and survival? These are some of the questions that this collection aims to answer.

Key themes

The chapters in this collection are unified by their attention to five key themes: the importance of regional and local perspectives; the formation and content of policy; the nature of activism; the role of international networks and exchange; and, finally, which histories are remembered, and how those processes of remembering and forgetting take place. These are all extremely important to the history of HIV/AIDS in particular, but many of the same questions, methods, and analytical frameworks in evidence here could be applied more broadly to histories of health and illness too.

The importance of national and regional circumstances to HIV/AIDS policy responses has long been acknowledged, not least because the emergence of this new and highly stigmatised disease seemed to draw particularly pointed attention to the political and cultural contexts in which decisions were made. Different countries followed different paths in their response. Early analyses noted a much greater reliance on mass testing and contact tracing in Sweden, for example, compared to the UK, where concerns about confidentiality and privacy meant that health education initiatives were preferred instead. These approaches also diverged from those of Spain and France, which saw an 'exclusive bio-medical emphasis', leaving matters in the hands of medical researchers, and from the 'more pragmatic approach in countries such as Holland, Denmark and Switzerland'.[32] The epidemiological picture also varied from place to place; in New York and Edinburgh, injecting drug use was understood to be a very common mode of HIV transmission, whereas elsewhere in the USA and UK the risk factor dominating official data was sex between men.[33] Inevitably, who was affected by HIV/AIDS and what they experienced as a result would vary dramatically, depending on location. Yet we still know relatively little about these differences and variations; within the dominant case study of the Anglo-American experience, regional variation is often smoothed over, and historical explorations of other geographical contexts are still relatively new.

Contributions to this collection are among the first sustained historical enquiries into HIV/AIDS in Norway, Italy, and Wales, while further chapters bring the Republic of Ireland, Switzerland, the Netherlands, Edinburgh, and briefly Germany and Poland into the mix as well. Insights from beyond the dominant Anglo-American historiography offer new approaches and issues; they draw attention to different concerns and different kinds of innovation in response to HIV/AIDS, to the involvement of different actors, and to relevant activist networks and interventions that pre-dated the emergence of HIV/AIDS. They also introduce new perspectives, situating European regions and nations in global contexts and highlighting matters of migration, criminalisation, and national myth-making. These ideas and approaches have played a lesser role in histories of HIV/AIDS in the UK and have something valuable to offer to those revisiting narratives focused on the UK (and USA).

Together, the chapters in this collection emphasise the role of national self-image, local and national epidemiology, and pre-existing structures, cultures, and practices in shaping how people and policies responded to HIV/AIDS, and, indeed, how it has been remembered. They also add nuance to the impression of panicked and hostile public reactions to the epidemic in the early years, soon overcome by science and sensible policy. Such reactions and policies are examined and carefully contextualised here. Panic and hostility were certainly present, but are not always found where they might be expected. Furthermore, many of the problems associated with the earlier years of the epidemic are far from resolved. Regional accounts, then, offer their own timelines, their own dominant actors, and their own emotional histories, at once familiar and unique.

Accounts of hostility or disinterest among policy-makers towards those affected by HIV/AIDS have been a common feature of popular histories of the epidemic. At their most simplistic, analyses of state policies relating to HIV/AIDS have portrayed them as either grossly reactionary and inadequate or overwhelmingly liberal and successful, depending on perspective. The authors here follow and develop more detailed explorations of policy-making in health and social care, drawing attention to factors such as perceptions of risk, international pressures, conflicting demands, influential individuals, and opportunities for rules and policies to be bent or broken. 'Official' responses to HIV/AIDS are also shown to extend far beyond pronouncements and public health messages from central government, for all that these kinds of interventions were important. Authoritative and significant responses to the crisis were also formulated in the offices of local governments, charities, specialist membership organisations, international bodies, and in the activities of social workers, researchers, clinicians, and curators too. Understanding the history of policy and practice surrounding HIV/AIDS, this collection suggests, demands attention to such efforts.

These approaches to HIV/AIDS might be characterised as 'top-down', involving organisations and individuals with a professional interest or responsibility. Yet, patient- and volunteer-led activism and action has long occupied a central position within histories of HIV/AIDS, and indeed more generally within histories of health and policy-making since the Second World War. HIV/AIDS has been connected to a broader shift in the idea of the expert, who was, by the end of the century, no longer always and only the doctor or other professional person. Expertise 'by experience' has become a well-known phrase, and the expert status that was eventually granted to (some) gay men during the HIV/AIDS crisis has been acknowledged as a feature of the early years of the epidemic in particular.

As the contributions to this collection begin to suggest, histories of HIV/AIDS have been distorted by this account in significant ways. In some quarters, and particularly where public health anxieties homed in on other groups such as sex workers or injecting drug users, the epidemic could prompt recognition of expertise among a wider constituency of people. However, as several chapters indicate, where multiple marginalised identities intersected, this recognition was only partial or temporary. Not all expertise by experience was equal. Nor was all activism successful and covered by the mainstream media. Local campaigns, covert activities, individual rule-breaking or boundary-testing, and other activities taking place behind the scenes, without eye-catching placards and slogans, profoundly affected policies and experiences. These kinds of activities are by their very nature harder to locate in more traditional archives and museum collections, which generally contain little about personal experience as opposed to official policy and research, and favour the successful and positive over the unpopular, failed, and fleeting. Yet, new archives and collections, along with efforts to ask new questions of older sources, can provide a much fuller picture of HIV/AIDS activism and expertise.

Expertise frequently drew on transnational networks, as individuals and groups worked hard to establish pathways for sharing information and ideas both within and beyond Western Europe. As the final two chapters of this volume clearly indicate, more varied resources for generating future histories will demand – and encourage – greater attention to international connections, global communities, and the porous nature of national borders when it comes to making sense of the complexities of HIV/AIDS. Activists, allies, and HIV/AIDS professionals travelled and read widely in search of insight and inspiration, although innovations from one region did not always translate easily elsewhere. International guidelines and standards, the business of international diplomacy, and national self-image all influenced policy, activism, and the networks that took shape. Some of these networks were initially short-lived, but many have had long afterlives.

Finally, this collection centres some of the cohorts of people who were greatly affected by HIV/AIDS, but who are still rarely mentioned in mainstream histories: sex workers, injecting drug users, gay men beyond the metropolis, women living with HIV, children, social workers, nurses, people in prison. Some chapters address the policies, anxieties, and activism that swirled around these groups, while others address more individual experiences. Archival gaps have been partially addressed through the generation and use of new oral histories but, clearly, many absences remain. There are particular gaps where multiple forms of marginalisation intersect: where drug users were also racialised, for example, or where women were also migrants. This issue comes to the fore in the final two chapters of the collection, which deal explicitly with questions of collecting and curating. How can the heterogeneous and sometimes conflicting memories and histories of HIV/AIDS be captured, created, sustained, and presented? Structural inequalities and marginalisation were so often at the heart of HIV/AIDS and are still very often embedded within the sources and stories in circulation. How can our future histories avoid reproducing this marginalisation and create fuller accounts of HIV/AIDS in the past?

Introducing the chapters

Marginalisation, its extent and its effects, is central to the chapter that opens this collection. Addressing HIV/AIDS policy in Norway with particular reference to sex workers, in Chapter 1 Ketil Slagstad and Anne Kveim Lie test the argument that HIV/AIDS created new constituents of experts who informed medicine and policy and delivered vital education. The inclusion of gay men as experts fitted well with the Norwegian self-image as a liberal, social-democratic state, but the inclusion of sex workers was not so easily achieved. Their chapter explores how and why sex workers came to be constituted as first a social problem and then a 'risk group' in Norway. Notably, sex workers were conceptualised as women who were a risk to others, and not as a group who were themselves at risk. Thanks in particular to the activities of social workers, a more nuanced understanding of sex work eventually emerged and the notions of listening to and learning from those involved, and of engaging in 'harm reduction' initiatives, prompted experiments in peer education and activism. Attention to harm reduction reflected the perceived and actual intersection between sex workers and drug users, while peer education was informed by initiatives abroad. Providing detailed insight into how officials and health workers in Norway dealt with HIV/AIDS, this chapter also listens to the words of sex workers interviewed in the midst of the crisis of the 1980s and early 1990s and more recently, speaking about their views and experiences.

Another marginalised group is central to Chapter 2 by Brian DeGrazia, on the opening of a centre for young HIV-positive drug users in Rome in 1988. Italy, like several other locations addressed in this collection, experienced an epidemic in which injecting drug use quickly became a primary epidemiological concern. Unsurprisingly, therefore, the rhetoric and policy surrounding drug use loomed large in the Italian response to HIV/AIDS. As this chapter shows, drug users were strongly associated with poverty and delinquency and public perceptions of HIV/AIDS – informed by public health messaging – were suffused with ideas of social contamination. Here, international influences are strongly in evidence in the form of American–Italian diplomatic relations and Italy's commitment to the American 'War on Drugs'. National self-image in another register is also important, with the idea of the traditional Italian family fuelling education campaigns and positioning drug users as 'beyond' the family unit. Here, also, is a more positive role for the Catholic Church than has typically been granted to religious bodies in relation to HIV/AIDS in the West – although their focus on caring for drug users, and not gay men affected by HIV/AIDS, is notable.

Low-profile and collaborative activism emerges in Chapter 3 by Janet Weston, on European prison policies surrounding HIV/AIDS. A comparative case study of the Republic of Ireland and Switzerland delivers one example of the role of local cultures and preoccupations in shaping policy. It also highlights two contrasting and little-known forms of activism in those countries, undertaken to try to protect the health of drug users in prisons. In Dublin, this was inspired by international networks and peer- and service user-led education, supported by social workers, and undertaken by prison officers, whereas in the Swiss context it was prison doctors who instigated change through private disobedience and public resignation, using professional medical standards to justify their actions. Contrasting local circumstances meant that these experiments met with rather different fates. As well as introducing this kind of activism to the history of HIV/AIDS, this chapter surveys prison policies relating to the epidemic across the Western European region, emphasising the important role of international guidelines and the specific areas of health promotion where prison priorities could not be reconciled with those of public health.

Chapter 4 returns to the better-known context of the UK in the 1980s and 1990s, but is the first of three chapters which begin to break this country up into its constituent nations. It uses newly gathered oral histories from nurses to explore experiences in a very particular location: HIV wards in hospitals in England. The paucity of information and biomedical solutions at first meant that HIV/AIDS prompted greater attention to the psychosocial elements of nursing care, although this was uneven and nurses struggled to balance this with enduring fear and uncertainty. As specialist HIV/AIDS nursing care developed, though, many queer nurses were drawn to the work, and HIV/AIDS wards could become spaces for camp humour and camaraderie. This raises important questions about who was included in these spaces and who was excluded, as does the question of patient expertise. Many nurses reported learning a great deal from their patients, but this kind of relationship was not replicated in all nursing contexts. This chapter reflects upon some of the complexities of the memories shared in oral history interviews and explores the sense of isolation or ostracisation that some nurses now remember, coupled with the potential (and desire) for rule-breaking and crafting new forms of care.

The limits of medical and social provision for people with HIV/AIDS in Wales is the subject of Daryl Leeworthy's Chapter 5, which highlights the impact on policy and public attitudes of the *absence* of a sense of crisis. In contrast to its closest neighbours England and Scotland, rates of HIV infection in Wales remained low and an impression lingered that this was not really a Welsh problem. Services were correspondingly patchy, especially outside of city centres. Financing and restructuring also presented consistent problems which continue to this day. Early efforts to develop locally tailored education programmes were designed with the perceived flaws of the British campaign in mind, and therefore focused to a great extent on positive information sharing, particularly with young people and medical professionals. Nevertheless, public opinion was complex and varied, with pockets of protest and fairly widespread homophobia. As in other chapters, new material is deployed here to inform our understanding of experiences of HIV/AIDS among gay and bisexual men, this time in the form of the telephone call logs of the Welsh telephone adviceline FRIEND in the 1980s and 1990s. This offers a particularly valuable snapshot of some of the emotions that swirled around HIV/AIDS for gay and bisexual men and their families.

Emotion plays a vital role in Hannah J. Elizabeth's Chapter 6, which moves the collection from Wales to Scotland and considers responses to mothers' medical, emotional and educational needs in particular. The relationship between mothers, their children, and the caring professions lies at the heart of the story here, as new services and spaces were developed for women affected by HIV/AIDS. These women were mainly injecting drug users, or the partners of drug users, and often had strained relationships with statutory services. Existing models of service provision would not work. As in Norway, it was health and social care workers who were prominent in the design and delivery of services, and their words, along with those of the women they worked with, are centred in this account. This chapter argues that the services and publications that emerged from Edinburgh should be seen as a form of activism, undertaken in true collaborative and interdisciplinary fashion but at risk of being forgotten. Close attention to new kinds of sources such as children's books, and revisiting more familiar types of text like newspaper reports and information leaflets with new eyes can help to capture experiences, activities, and attitudes that might otherwise disappear.

The final two chapters of this collection return to the question of how the crisis of the 1980s and 1990s is, and can be, remembered. They reflect on the processes through which HIV/AIDS archives and museum collections are gathered and made available, and challenge us to consider the impact and future of such efforts. Chapter 7, from the writing and research team behind the European HIV/AIDS Archive (EHAA), situates this archive in the context of challenges and tensions surrounding the production of memories and histories of HIV/AIDS. The response of the authors is to theorise the EHAA as a form of 'queer counter-memory', in which contradictions and disappointments, ambiguities and uncertainties, exclusions and absences are all foregrounded. Through the selection of interview subjects, the mode of interviewing, the choices surrounding metadata and archival boundaries, and the presentation of an archive that is incomplete and subject to change, the EHAA becomes not only an immensely useful resource for researchers, but also a vehicle for reflecting on the uneasy, conflicting, and complex histories and futures of HIV/AIDS.

To conclude the collection, in Chapter 8 Manon S. Parry addresses the role of museums in conveying the complexity and diversity of HIV/AIDS histories. Prompted by the 2018 International AIDS Society conference in Amsterdam and the cultural activities surrounding it, this final chapter considers the history of museum exhibits about HIV/AIDS. It pays particular attention to the ways in which national contexts and cultures combine with specific museum practices to restrict the items that can be, or have been, collected. This, in turn, restricts the stories that can be told in exhibitions about HIV/AIDS. The case study of one exhibition on display in Amsterdam during the 2018 conference reveals a positive nationalistic narrative, focusing on white gay men, in which Dutch tolerance and liberalism along with scientific innovation and influential individuals eventually leads to success in bringing HIV/AIDS in the Netherlands under control. This is contrasted at the end of the exhibition with ongoing crises overseas. By saying little about the role of structural inequalities, about other communities affected by HIV/AIDS, including women, drug users, migrants, and those with haemophilia, about global connections, or about ongoing domestic issues in terms of rising HIV infection rates and stigma, public histories such as this remain partial and problematic.

These questions about who and what is included in exhibitions, archives, and historical narratives, shaping how pandemics are understood and remembered, are essential to this collection. Many of the chapters here were written before the emergence of Covid-19, but the collection was compiled under its shadow and Parry's chapter concludes with reflections on some of the lessons from HIV/AIDS for those concerned with capturing histories of present and future pandemics. The stories we tell about the past have real present-day impact; glossing over its ambiguities and complexities has particular ramifications for those whose lives are situated at the heart of these complexities. And, although this collection strives to present a wider range of histories that includes previously marginalised voices and often overlooked experiences, we are acutely aware that many histories are still excluded. As a number of chapters acknowledge, many of these investigations are only beginning to scratch the surface. More nuanced insights that take into account multiple identities and multiple forms of marginalisation, geographic mobilities, structural inequalities, and the roles of racism, nationalism, and ideas of citizenship within histories of HIV/AIDS are still needed. Additional oral histories, along with expanding and increasingly diverse archives and the attention of more historians as well as scholars from other disciplines, will help to bring this into being.

This collection has its origins in a workshop held at Birkbeck, University of London, in July 2018, as part of the month-long AIDS Histories and Cultures Festival convened by the Raphael Samuel History Centre. Initially designated as a workshop to consider histories of HIV/AIDS across Europe as a whole, it quickly became apparent that our geographical coverage was extremely patchy. The regional focus of this collection, where Northern Europe and particularly the UK dominates, reflects the historiography and history of HIV/AIDS to date, as well as the availability of archival materials and the fact of this being published in English. With relatively little work in English on non–Anglo-American histories of HIV/AIDS, there has also been limited scope here for exploring comparisons and connections across regions and nations. No doubt such explorations will, when they become possible, situate Europe more fully within its global and (post)colonial setting.

Although this collection introduces only a small selection of under-examined regions, nations, populations, individuals, archives, and issues, we hope that it will prompt new questions and approaches, encouraging rich histories of HIV/AIDS in the future. This collection can serve as a starting point and inspiration for further research in these directions, and may help to sustain an interest in more integrated, transnational, and intersectional histories of HIV/AIDS within and beyond Western Europe. There are already inspiring signs of this, in the form of work that is starting to fill some of the geographical and conceptual gaps in this collection. Current research into histories of HIV/AIDS in France, Spain, Denmark, and Germany, countries notable in their absence here, is beginning to build a fuller picture of the Western European context. Central, Eastern, and pan-European explorations are also beginning to appear, offering invaluable insights into policies and experiences of HIV/AIDS within different cultural and political settings, playing out across different time frames. Importantly, this research is recognising the importance of the local and global as well as the national, and is drawing on a wide array of newly collected and previously unused source material.[34] We look forward to this renaissance of HIV/AIDS histories with great enthusiasm, and hope that this collection will contribute in some small way to its diversity, scope, and ambition.

Notes

1 Chris Beyrer, 'A pandemic anniversary: 40 years of HIV/AIDS', *The Lancet*, 397.10290 (2021), 2142–3.

2 These include memorials or monuments in Frankfurt (unveiled in 1994), Barcelona (2003), Vancouver (2004), Moscow (2004), Vienna (2007), Tenerife (2008), Belarus (2008), Brighton (2009), Seville (2015), New York (2016), West Hollywood (scheduled to open in late 2022), and many more; exhibitions of memorial quilts across and beyond Europe and the USA; developing collections and recent exhibitions at museums including Mucem in Marseille, the Schwules Museum in Berlin, and the online UK HIV/AIDS Design Archive (www.hivgraphiccommunication.com, accessed 10 October 2021), and reflections on these including Florent Molle, 'Construire une exposition sur l'histoire sociale du VIH-sida au Mucem', *La lettre de l'OCIM*, 183 (2019), https://doi.org/10.4000/ocim.2473 (accessed 10 October 2021); Theodore (ted) Kerr, 'What you don't know about AIDS could fill a museum: curatorial ethics and the ongoing epidemic in the 21st century', *On Curating*, 42 (2019), 5–13.

3 We and the contributors to this collection use the term 'HIV/AIDS' throughout, except where referring specifically to either HIV or AIDS. Although HIV and AIDS are now recognised as distinct medical conditions, they have been much confused and conflated over the last forty years, and policy responses and activism have both often tackled them as one and the same issue.

4 See the articles about AIDS in *Annals of Internal Medicine*, 98:3 (March 1983), 277–303 discussing Kaposi's Sarcoma among Haitians and cases of AIDS among patients with haemophilia.
5 World Health Organization, *AIDS prevention and control: invited presentations and papers from the World Summit of Ministers of Health on Programmes for AIDS Prevention* (Geneva; Oxford: World Health Organization; Pergamon Press, 1988), p. 28.
6 Global Commission on HIV and the Law, *High income countries issue brief: laws and practices related to criminalisation of people living with HIV and populations vulnerable to HIV* (New York: United Nations Development Programme, 2011), pp. 12–13.
7 Srdan Matic, Jeffrey V. Lazarus, and Martin C. Donoghoe (eds), *HIV/AIDS in Europe: moving from death sentence to chronic disease management* (Copenhagen: World Health Organization Europe, 2006), pp. 1, 6.
8 UNAIDS, *The changing HIV/AIDS epidemic in Europe and Central Asia* (Geneva: Joint United Nations Programme on HIV/AIDS, 2004), pp. 7–9.
9 UNAIDS, *UNAIDS data 2020* (Geneva: Joint United Nations Programme on HIV/AIDS, 2020), p. 378, available online at www.unaids.org/en/resources/documents/2020/unaids-data (accessed 10 January 2021).
10 Randy Shilts, *And the band played on: politics, people, and the AIDS epidemic* (New York: St. Martin's Press, 1987); Dennis Altman, *AIDS and the new puritanism* (London: Pluto Press, 1986); Douglas Crimp (ed.), *AIDS: cultural analysis, cultural activism*, 1st edn (Cambridge, MA: MIT Press, 1988); Peter Aggleton, Graham Hart, and Peter Davies (eds), *AIDS: social representations, social practices* (New York: Falmer Press, 1989).
11 Allan M. Brandt, *No magic bullet: a social history of venereal disease in the United States since 1880*, expanded edn (New York; Oxford: Oxford University Press, 1987); Frank Mort, *Dangerous sexualities: medico-moral politics in England since 1830* (London: Routledge & Kegan Paul, 1987); Jeffrey Weeks, *Coming out: homosexual politics in Britain from the nineteenth century to the present*, revised edn (London: Quartet, 1990).
12 Cindy Patton, *Last served?: Gendering the HIV pandemic* (London; Bristol, PA: Taylor & Francis, 1994).
13 Roy Porter, 'History says no to the policeman's response to AIDS', *British Medical Journal*, 293.6562 (1986), 1589–90.

14 Elizabeth Fee and Daniel M. Fox (eds), *AIDS: the making of a chronic disease* (Berkeley, CA: University of California Press, 1992).
15 Jeffrey Weeks, 'AIDS: the intellectual agenda', in *AIDS: social representations, social practices*, ed. by Peter Aggleton, Graham Hart, and Peter Davies (New York: Falmer Press, 1989), pp. 1–20; Eric T. Juengst and Barbara A. Koenig (eds), *The meaning of AIDS: implications for medical science, clinical practice, and public health policy* (New York: Praeger, 1989); Davinia Cooper, 'Off the banner and onto the agenda: the emergence of a new municipal lesbian and gay politics, 1979–86', *Critical Social Policy*, 12.36 (1993), 20–39.
16 Jonathan Zimmerman, *Too hot to handle: a global history of sex education* (Oxford: Princeton University Press, 2015).
17 Fee and Fox (eds), *AIDS: the making of a chronic disease*; Virginia Berridge, *AIDS in the UK: the making of policy, 1981–1994* (Oxford: Oxford University Press, 1996); Patton, *Last served?*.
18 Kerr, 'What you don't know about AIDS could fill a museum'.
19 A small selection includes *How to Survive a Plague* (dir. David France, 2012, and associated book published in 2016); *United in Anger* (dir. Jim Hubbard, 2012); *The Dallas Buyers Club* (dir. Jean-Marc Vallée, 2013); Alysia Abbot, *Fairyland: a memoir of my father* (London: W. W. Norton, 2013); Cynthia Carr, *Fire in the belly: the life and times of David Wojnarowicz* (New York: Bloomsbury, 2013); *Art AIDS America* (New York: The Bronx Museum of the Arts, 2016); *AIDS in New York: The first five years* (New York: New York Historical Society, 2013); *120 battements par minute* (dir. Robin Campillo, 2017); *Epidemic: When Britain Fought Aids* (Channel 4, 2017).
20 An early example is Victoria Angela Harden, *AIDS at 30: a history*, (Washington, DC: Potomac Books, 2012). See also Helen Coyle, 'A tale of one city: a history of HIV/AIDS policy-making in Edinburgh, 1982–1994' (unpublished PhD thesis, University of Edinburgh, 2008).
21 Richard A. McKay, *Patient Zero and the making of the AIDS epidemic* (Chicago, IL: University of Chicago Press, 2017); 'HIV/AIDS and U.S. History', *Journal of American History*, 104.2 (2017), 431–60.
22 Christophe Broqua, *Action=vie: a history of AIDS activism and gay politics in France* (Philadelphia, PA: Temple University Press, 2020); Elisabet Björklund and Mariah Larsson (eds), *A visual history of HIV/AIDS: exploring The Face of AIDS Film Archive* (Abingdon: Routledge, 2018).
23 Mary Kenny, 'When youth went to pot', *Daily Mail*, 2 June 1987, p. 21.

24 Alan Hamilton, 'Singing was just a ploy to get noticed and get boys', *The Sunday Times*, 4 May 1991, p. 56.
25 See Jock Young, 'Moral panic: its origins in resistance, ressentiment and the translation of fantasy into reality', *British Journal of Criminology*, 49.1 (2009), 4–16.
26 Emma Forrest, 'Sung from the heart', *The Sunday Times*, 19 September 1993, pp. 9–10.
27 Graham Turner, 'City of a million sorrows: Britain must heed the lessons of New York's slide into an abyss of drugs and violence', *Daily Mail*, 6 November 1989, pp. 20–1.
28 Thomson Prentice, 'Nightmare of a raddled city', *The Times*, 29 October 1986, p. 14.
29 Ann Leslie, 'Nightmare needle park: overdose that killed drugs colony', *Daily Mail*, 17 February 1992, pp. 6–7.
30 William Davies, 'Double curse of the AIDS plague city: the drugs were bad enough… now the addicts' needles are creating a horror on a unique scale behind Edinburgh's elegant façade', *Daily Mail*, 11 April 1986, p. 6.
31 *Ibid*.
32 Daniel M. Fox, Patricia Day, and Rudolf Klein, 'The power of professionalism: policies for AIDS in Britain, Sweden, and the United States', *Daedalus*, 118.2 (1989), 93–112; Simon Watney, *Practices of freedom: selected writings on HIV/AIDS* (Durham, NC: Duke University Press, 1994), pp. 84–5, 154.
33 J. R. Robertson, A. B. Bucknall, P. D. Welsby, J. J. Roberts, J. M. Inglis, J. F. Peutherer, and R. P. Brettle, 'Epidemic of AIDS related virus (HTLV-III/LAV) infection among intravenous drug abusers', *British Medical Journal*, 292.6519 (1986), 527–9.
34 Examples of this burgeoning work include the CHAD project at the University of Copenhagen, running from August 2021 to December 2024; Aimar Olabarria Arriola, 'Animals, touch, and books: surface matters in the HIV/AIDS archive' (unpublished PhD thesis, Goldsmiths, University of London, 2020); Renaud Chantraine, Florent Molle, and Sandrine Musso, 'AIDS politics of representation and narratives: a current project at the Museum of European and Mediterranean Civilizations in Marseille, France', *On Curating*, 42 (2019), 206–18; Friederike Faust, 'The prisoner citizen: juridification and the AIDS activist struggle for harm reduction in German prisons', *Critical Public Health*, 31.1 (2021), 17–29; Johanna Folland, 'Globalizing socialist health: Africa, East Germany, and the AIDS crisis' (unpublished PhD thesis, University of Michigan, 2019); Patrick

McDonagh, *Gay and lesbian activism in the Republic of Ireland, 1973–93* (London: Bloomsbury, 2021). See also forthcoming work by Kateřina Kolářová on the politics of HIV/AIDS in the Czech Republic, Chase Ledin on representations of AIDS since 1996, George Severs on HIV/AIDS activism in England, and Louie Dean Valencia-García on HIV/AIDS policy and community in Europe.

1

Selling sex in the age of HIV/AIDS: activism, politics, and medicine in Norway, 1983–90

Ketil Slagstad and Anne Kveim Lie

HIV/AIDS was from the beginning a heavily politicised disease.[1] The epidemic exposed conflicting value systems and disagreements within science, medicine, public health, and clinical practice. It raised challenges to the power of doctors to privilege some while marginalising others, and it exposed how medicine constructs boundaries. The construction of 'risk groups' by classical epidemiology, carried out by public health practitioners and policy-makers, is a case in point. In this chapter, we follow the construction of one such risk group, 'prostitutes'.[2] On one hand, the response to HIV/AIDS followed the trajectory of a traditional blame game; on the other, it also gave voice to those affected by the epidemic.

Little has been written about Norwegian HIV/AIDS history in general and about sex work and HIV/AIDS in particular.[3] This chapter draws on a range of material from public and private archives, as well as oral history interviews with activists and civil servants, to explore this history. We begin with the emergence of prostitution as a 'social problem' in Norway and then discuss the construction of sex workers as a 'risk group' within the epidemic. Becoming a risk group meant posing a risk to the public, but not being recognised as a group of people with their own health risks and needs. It took a long time before authorities and outreach services began to recognise how diverse sex workers were, facing intersecting forms of marginalisation in relation to gender, class, and space. Finally, we discuss an attempt by the Norwegian health authorities to include women who sold sex as health promoters among their peers.

The inclusion of gay and lesbian activists in public HIV/AIDS work fitted well with the philosophy of the welfare state and Norwegian public health traditions. But it was much more controversial among authorities, social workers, politicians, and the police to include sex workers in a similar way. In the early 1980s, political parties agreed that prostitution was an unwanted phenomenon, and in public health and in the press the (female) sex worker was portrayed as a reservoir of infection and vector for HIV transmission. As the epidemic unfolded, however, it was increasingly realised that people who sold sex were a heterogeneous group with differing health needs. Subsequent public health approaches increasingly aimed to mitigate the fact that sex workers were themselves at risk, and some prevention strategies included activists and people who sold sex. Ultimately, HIV/AIDS gave impetus to early sex worker activism. Today, activists continue to oppose the criminalisation of sex work and call for the inclusion of sex workers in harm-reduction policy. The story of Norway's HIV/AIDS crisis shows how public health policy can reinforce the stigmatisation of sex workers, but also how inclusion and collaboration can promote effective public health interventions.

Prostitution becomes a social problem

In a study of Norwegian media coverage of prostitution, sociologist May-Len Skilbrei showed that the press in the 1970s did not usually present prostitution as a problem.[4] Prostitution was discussed either as an exotic phenomenon or a nuisance to the public, but this changed towards the end of the decade. As a part of a more general trend to problematise an increasingly wide range of social practices, prostitution came to be seen as a social problem to be amended by social and political means. A first sign of this change was when minors selling sex in downtown Oslo became the focus of discussion in 1977–8.[5] Feminists turned their attention to this, seeing it as the result of patriarchy, the exploitation of women and girls, and structural gender-based discrimination in society.[6] This contributed to making prostitution a visible social problem, and the feminists' solution was police reporting, rallies, and militant actions. For example, in the early 1980s, radical feminists painted 'whoremonger' [horekunde] on cars in central Oslo where women sold sex – with the media in tow.[7] The focus had gradually shifted from 'hookers' and pimps to buyers and wider society. In the 1980s, the media increasingly turned to the life stories of sex workers themselves.[8] The 1982 autobiography of 'Ida' entitled *Hard Asfalt* ('hard asphalt'), in which she described her tragic story of being forced to sell sex to pay for her drug use, sold 70,000 copies in just a few months. Prostitution was increasingly seen as harmful to the women involved.

While feminists were fighting prostitution through militant activism, social work interventions were increasingly called for instead. This was part of a more general trend in Norway, where the relatively new profession of social work became the platform for government intervention in social problems.[9] Public attention led to the establishment of the 'Oslo project', a two-year social service programme run by sociologists and social workers aimed at mapping the extent of 'child and youth prostitution' in the capital and helping minors to find alternatives.[10] The project served as a starting point for later social work initiatives with women of all ages selling sex throughout Norway.[11]

The project put prostitution on the political agenda. In the same year, a special unit was set up with the Oslo police to make it easier for sex workers to obtain police help. Prostitution was not criminalised, but a 'pimp paragraph' in the criminal law prohibited the running of brothels or renting of premises for prostitution. Moreover, sex workers were not allowed to work in public spaces.[12] This legislation dated back to changes to Norwegian law in the very early twentieth century to regulate prostitution by prohibiting loitering and procurement.[13] In the early 1980s, a proposal to criminalise sexual services more directly was not taken up by the Ministry of Justice, partly for fear of driving prostitution underground and further harming those who sold sex.[14]

In August 1983, a shelter was established for women who sold sex in Oslo. This represented a completely new way of dealing with prostitution as a social and political issue. The goal was to 'rehabilitate' women who sold sex,[15] and the Oslo project enjoyed broad support across political parties, and with feminists across party lines.[16] Since the shelter also served women outside of the capital and because of its radically new approach, funding was secured not only from the City of Oslo, but also from the Ministry of Social Affairs. The shelter had space for thirteen people in three flats and was run by social workers from the beginning. This shelter later became the Pro Centre, a social service centre offering help and care for sex workers and advocating for sex workers' rights which still exists today. The Oslo project, the shelter, and later the Pro Centre were the foundation of social work for people who sold sex in Norway.

As support services for sex workers were formalised in the 1980s, social workers came into close contact with women selling sex. Gradually, the Pro Centre expanded its services and changed its focus. It had started as a shelter to help those seeking alternative livelihoods, but soon also included walk-in services, individual therapy, and weekly meetings where sex workers could talk openly about their life problems. One of the regular meetings was meant to empower women to 'talk about what it means to be a woman'.[17] It became clear that many sex workers shared some characteristics. Many came from deprived backgrounds, many used drugs, and most had very limited employment opportunities.[18] Social workers and activists realised that the women who used their services often suffered from 'big emotional problems' and needed a long period of rehabilitation and follow-up after they left.[19] Others needed help finding jobs, enrolling in education programmes, or finding housing. This realisation prompted social workers to steer work at the acute shelter away from the traditional social work philosophy and in a more 'therapeutic direction'.[20] The centre had identified an unmet need for psychological and medical services among people selling sex. Even though the shelter did not directly provide medical services, it worked with rehabilitation services, doctors, and hospitals, to which social workers would refer women who sold sex.[21] Gradually, prostitution became not only a social problem, but also a *medical* one.

The arrival of AIDS: sex workers become a risk group

If the early 1980s can be seen as the beginning of the medicalisation of sex work in Norway, the emergence of HIV/AIDS catalysed this development. The 1970s with its sexual revolution and women's rights movements had brought the rights of sexual minorities and women to the centre stage of public discourse. However, many people saw these changes as a sign that society was drifting in unwanted directions and breaking with Christian values and traditional ideas of the nuclear family.[22] HIV/AIDS emerged into this complex context, where progressive experiments co-existed with conservative reaction.[23] In many countries, the epidemic was used as an opportunity to challenge the recent liberalisation of society and promote conservative values. HIV/AIDS was portrayed by many as being not first and foremost a biomedical issue, but a moral crisis caused by certain sexual identities or practices.[24] Prevention therefore meant prescribing moral behaviour.

In 1983, the first patients were diagnosed with AIDS in Norway. The same year, the director general of health, Torbjørn Mork, established a working group on acquired immune deficiencies. The group was to coordinate surveillance of the epidemic in Norway and stay up to date on scientific findings and the international epidemiological situation. As in most other countries, preventive work was from the outset focused on certain 'risk groups'. The concept of the AIDS risk group arose from the initial efforts of the United States Centers for Disease Control (CDC) to specify 'subgroups' at risk of developing AIDS. The original risk group, homosexuals, was soon joined by Haitians, heroin addicts, and haemophiliacs, forming the '4 Hs'.[25] But designating risk groups concealed the fact that it was not sexual identity, nationality, or the use of drugs per se that was responsible for the transmission of the virus, but the exchange of bodily fluids. Defining entire groups as being 'at risk' made it possible to separate these groups from the rest of the population. As historians of disease have argued, such an attribution of sexually transmitted disease to the 'cultural other' predates the formation of risk groups for HIV/AIDS by hundreds of years.[26]

In the first official circular sent to hospitals in April 1983, the Norwegian authorities copied the American model; the groups at risk [smittefaregrupper] were defined as 'sex partners of AIDS patients, sexually active homosexual and bisexual men with many sex partners, current and former injecting drug users, Haiti immigrants, patients with haemophilia and sex partners of people with high risk of infection'.[27] The cause of AIDS was unknown, but the circular stated that it was highly likely that it was caused by an infectious agent, and that transmission was similar to hepatitis B either through 'intimate contact or blood transfusion'.[28] The attention was focused on people in these risk groups, who were also asked to refrain from donating blood. Prevention work towards what was considered the main risk group, homosexual and bisexual men, was initiated by lesbian and gay activists who established the Gay Health Committee [*Helseutvalget for homofile*] in 1983.[29]

Early in the epidemic, there were already reports about heterosexual transmission,[30] but it would take some years before it was fully acknowledged that sexual transmission was not confined to homosexual and bisexual men. In 1985 and 1986, heterosexual transmission was still much debated in international medical journals, especially whether men could be infected by women.[31] Paula A. Treichler has argued that it was not until 1986 that the American HIV/AIDS epidemic became 'diversified'; until then, it had mostly been perceived as a homosexual epidemic. Treichler interpreted this shift as the result not of groundbreaking new insights into transmission mechanisms, but of a change in how facts were used and how HIV/AIDS was framed and understood.[32] The increased focus on heterosexual transmission led to the targeting of a new risk group: female sex workers. As the epidemic was diversified, this meant a shift not only in terms of sexuality but also gender; women increasingly became the risk group. In the director general of health's programme for AIDS, released in 1985, the risk groups, now defined as 'groups at high risk of contagion' [*høysmittefaregrupper*], had changed. Haitians were no longer seen as a threat (not surprising, since there were hardly any Haitian immigrants in Norway), but a new group had been added, namely, 'prostitutes'.[33]

Initially, 'prostitutes' were seen primarily as a danger to the rest of the population rather than as being at risk themselves.[34] In August 1985, for example, the head physician of the Oslo clinic for sexually transmitted infections expressed the view that sex workers 'will be the really big challenge to the AIDS problem in the years to come'.[35] In his opinion, sex workers had an increased risk of contracting HIV because of their weak immune systems. These 'girls', he warned, were likely to be irresponsible transmitters of the disease, who 'would probably use their seropositivity as an excuse to get more drugs'.[36] Concomitantly in the international medical debate, sex workers were portrayed as contaminated bodies harbouring large volumes of microbes. In 1985 in the *Journal of the American Medical Association*, for instance, it was reported that '[p]rostitutes could serve as a reservoir for HTLV-III infection for heterosexually active individuals'.[37] Gay men had been perceived as a relatively well-confined risk group that did not pose any risk to the wider public as a 'reservoir of infection'. Sex workers were presented as a completely different situation.

The authorities increasingly saw the heterosexual population as being at risk. When the first action plan against HIV was released in 1986, high-risk groups were defined as men who had sex with men, people who injected drugs, prostitutes, and people with sex partners from certain parts of the world. In addition, sex partners of people in the 'risk groups' were at risk, as well as people who regularly received blood products.[38] In a circular about the prevention and control of HIV/AIDS published by the Directorate of Health only six months later, sexual transmission was addressed in much more detail and the circular underscored that HIV could be transmitted through 'sexual contact from man to man, from man to woman, and from woman to man'.[39] Information campaigns were directed not only at designated risk groups, but also at the 'general' population. This broader perception of risk contributed to new public health goals. In its programme for HIV/AIDS in 1988, the Directorate of Health had two main ambitions: to prevent the spread of HIV and to prevent 'negative consequences of the HIV epidemic'.[40] Such negative consequences included unnecessary anxiety, marginalisation of risk groups, and scapegoating and discrimination; 'it has been and will be of major importance to avoid these attitudes'.[41]

The arrival of antibody tests also contributed to this change. Some tests for the HTLV-III virus had been available at specialist centres from the end of 1984, but it was not until spring 1985 that antibody testing became commercially available, in Norway as elsewhere. The Director General of Health's working group on HIV/AIDS advised that public health officials should address the general population regularly about risk factors, who should get tested, and where. Counselling and information were to be targeted at high-risk groups, but it was also important to reach 'everyone who is sexually active and everyone who is about to have sex for the first time'.⁴² Although mass testing had shown encouraging results, officials were more and more worried about heterosexual transmission.⁴³ The shift in transmission pattern was primarily seen among people who had sex with people in the risk groups. Sexual transmission through prostitution had not been noticed in Norway, but people who had bought sex abroad had been infected.

The change in nomenclature in the mid-1980s from 'homosexual/bisexual men' to 'men who have sex with men' was indicative of the gradual shift away from focusing on cultural groups and identities, towards specifying risky practices instead. But this change did not affect those who sold sex; female 'prostitutes' were still seen as a confined and defined cultural group that posed a risk to everyone else. In the 1986 book *AIDS – en utfordring til oss alle* [*AIDS – a challenge to us all*] a Norwegian infectious disease specialist and expert on HIV/AIDS told men to completely refrain from having sex with prostitutes, but did not think it important to warn sex workers of the risk of infection.⁴⁴ Prejudices and political resistance stood in the way of a destigmatising approach to sex workers, similar to that which had been developed for other marginalised groups.

Media spectacle and AIDS: 'the prostitute' as vector

In mid-1985, a left-liberal newspaper published a series of articles on the role of sex workers in the epidemic; 'AIDS among Oslo hookers' stood in big letters on the front page, as shown in Figure 1.1. After one of the women who sold sex tested positive, 'the alarm had been sounded in Oslo prostitution circles'. The passive grammatical construction gave no information about *who* had sounded the alarm.⁴⁵ A whole page was devoted to the topic, under an ominous title with strong war metaphors; 'I am a living death machine', the heading read, referring to the self-description of an HIV-positive woman selling sex (see Figure 1.2). Readers got to know twenty-five-year-old 'Bente', who was 'full of poison and spreads death and destruction' to finance her drug use. The positive test had completely changed her life. 'We are treated like lepers', she told the journalist, explaining that other sex workers wanted people like her off the streets, because they scared away the customers. Now, they had a hard time finding places to live or work. Reflecting

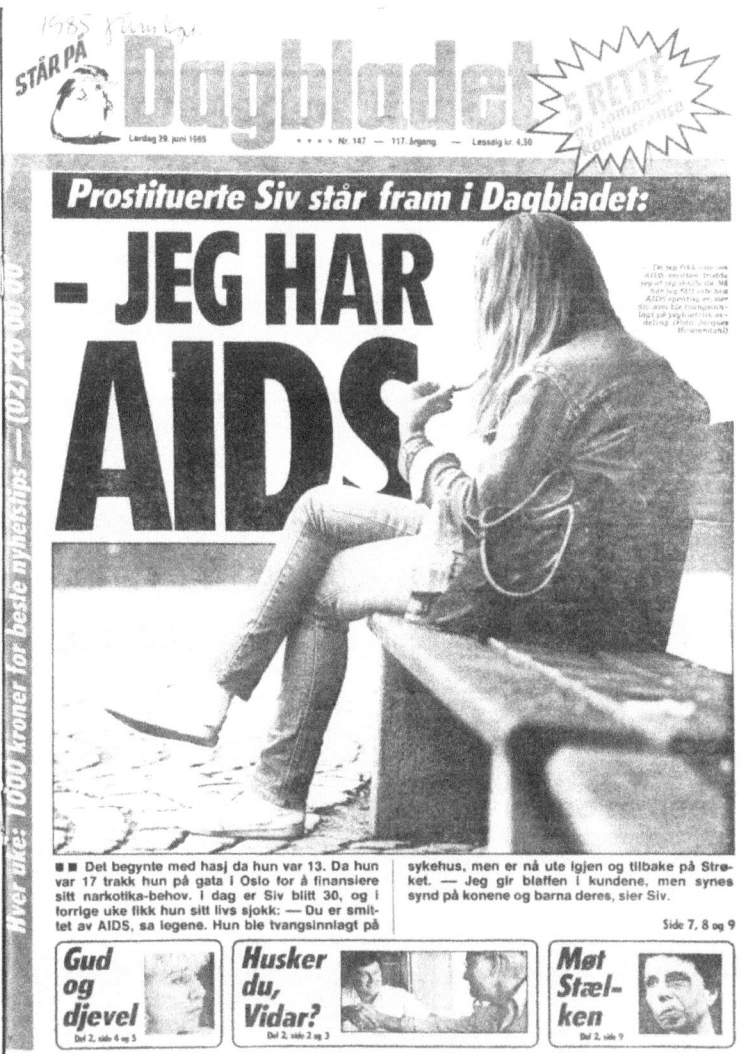

Figure 1.1 Facsimile from *Dagbladet*, 29 June 1985. The notion of prostitutes as vectors of AIDS was cemented by a series of newspaper articles. On the front page of this newspaper it said in bold letters: 'Siv, the prostitute, comes out in Dagbladet – I have AIDS'. (Copyright: *Dagbladet*)

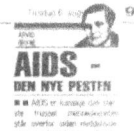

Figure 1.2 Facsimile from *Dagbladet*, 6 August 1985. 'I am a living death machine'. The press not only portrayed sex workers in a dehumanising way; the descriptions were even taken up by sex workers themselves.
(Copyright: *Dagbladet*)

menstrual taboos long preceding the HIV/AIDS epidemic,[46] one of the interviewees related that menstrual blood was associated with contamination: 'If menstruation blood gets on the bed sheets or in the shower, everything needs to be disinfected. That's why we are not accepted in any guesthouses.'[47]

The antibody tests made it possible for a person to be identified as a 'death machine'; self-stigma even made people take up these words to describe themselves. But the identification of the female 'prostitute body' as a vector or even reservoir of infection, transmitting an epidemic to the 'general population', has a long history.[48] Marie Spongberg, in her study of nineteenth-century prostitution, showed that aetiological theories of spontaneous generation of disease within the female sexual organs played an important role in campaigns to discipline people who sold sex.[49] Female sexual organs, especially those of 'prostitutes', were associated with disease and decay. In Norway from 1842, women who sold sex or were suspected of doing so had to appear regularly for medical inspections at the police doctor's office. Every eighth or fourteenth day, sex workers had to be certified as disease-free, and if they were suspected of being infected they were admitted to a hospital. So dominant was this view of women as the containers of the 'virus' that the need to examine customers was not addressed.[50] The medical goal of combating venereal disease in the nineteenth century was thus intertwined with gendered understandings of different sexual needs between men and women in general, and misogynistic notions of women in prostitution in particular.[51]

During the HIV/AIDS epidemic, sex workers faced similar gendered prejudices and biases. In several countries, restrictive legal measures like compulsory testing of sex workers were introduced.[52] Women who sold sex were seen as merely causal agents, spreading infection to the 'general population'. Women with HIV/AIDS were scapegoated as vectors of infection and were not seen as humans who were at risk of HIV themselves, as people who potentially were in need of health services.[53] In the Norwegian press, sex workers were often portrayed in a dehumanising and misogynist manner and referred to as 'AIDS hookers', as shown in Figure 1.3.[54] Newspapers also addressed the alleged risk to the most vulnerable segment of the population: children. Some of the customers' 'new, fancy cars' had children's safety seats installed, one newspaper

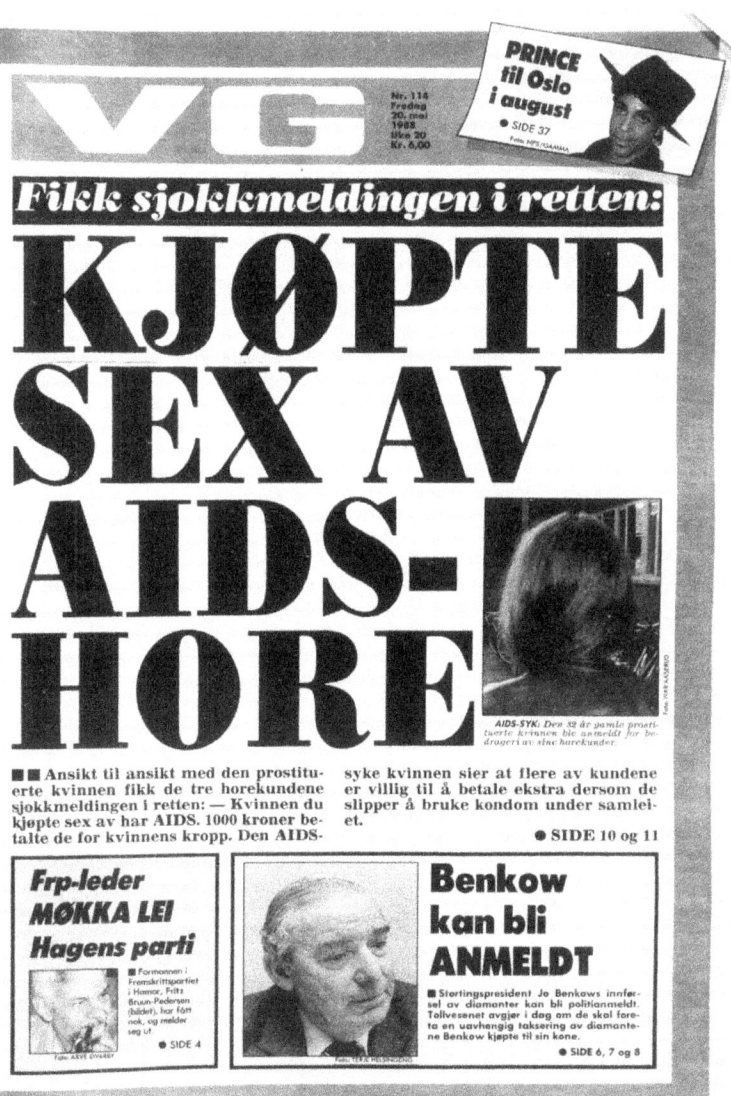

Figure 1.3 Facsimile from *VG*, 20 May 1988. 'Bought sex from AIDS hooker'. Sex workers living with HIV or AIDS were repeatedly referred to as 'AIDS hookers' in newspapers in the 1980s. (Copyright: *VG*)

reported.⁵⁵ This reflects a trope within newspaper coverage of the epidemic at that time; infants, haemophiliacs, and people who had blood transfusions were consistently referred to as 'innocent' victims. By implication, other people living with HIV/AIDS were guilty and worthy of blame. As Susan Sontag reminded us, 'innocence, by the inexorable logic that governs all relational terms, suggests guilt'.⁵⁶ Newspaper articles emphasised the risk that sex workers posed to the heterosexual 'general population' during the epidemic, and especially to innocent wives and children at home, implying that sex workers and customers alike were not only guilty, but also clearly *not* a part of this 'general population'.

Sex workers themselves vocalised concern about these 'innocent victims'. Siv, for instance, a thirty-year-old woman, told the newspaper that she always used condoms with customers. '[K]issing those pigs was never an option … I hate them. To be honest, I really don't care if I've infected them. They don't deserve any better', she said. 'What worries me are the families. The wives and kids who don't have an idea what's going on'.⁵⁷ Here, Siv disrupted the prevailing narrative of the sex worker as vector by emphasising her use of condoms and highlighting the client's role in transmission.⁵⁸ However, to some extent she also accepted the stereotypes of innocent and, by extension, guilty participants. Even though sex workers like Siv made it clear that they took precautions and used condoms, the notion of sex workers fuelling the epidemic and spreading it to the respectable majority was still disseminated. In the years that followed, the threat that HIV posed to the general population was discussed more and more, cementing the myth of sex workers as important vectors of transmission.

Sex workers as a public health risk

In the late 1980s, a series of research projects were conducted by public health officials on sex work and HIV/AIDS. These studies contributed to the perception that sex workers were a high-risk group. In 1987, the Norwegian Institute of Public Health began conducting studies to investigate the potential risk that sex workers posed by spreading HIV/AIDS. One study that looked at condom use among customers found that although half of all customers used condoms when buying sex, they did not also use them with other sex partners.[59] The study is a perfect example of how morality and science have been mixed up. By labelling men who bought sex as 'unfaithful', the researchers situated them in relation to their domestic, heterosexual relationships and reduced sex workers to vessels of contagion by presenting the transmission of HIV as unidirectional – from 'the prostitute' via customers to the 'general population'. This was also underscored by the research project title, 'Condom use among prostitutes', although the study subjects were actually their clients.

Another study looked at the health of sex workers and the risk they posed to public health. The objective of the study was to protect society.[60] At that time, the police had registered around 600 persons selling sex in Oslo, and some of the findings from the study must have been well-known facts to people working with sex workers: an overrepresentation of women who had experienced difficult childhoods, traumatising life events, and sexualised violence at a young age. Half of the women had injected drugs. Importantly, the study revealed that sex workers were generally open and positive about HIV testing; only five women refused to get tested. Many had been tested several times, often out of concern for others. 'It's better to know for sure than not knowing. I have so many around me I need to show regard for', one woman said. Another said that it's 'not like I can go around killing people'.[61] All used condoms; there were only a handful of incidents where the customer had not used a condom. Some customers paid extra for sex without a condom; some women found it difficult to refuse when customers asked for this; others had a trusting relationship with the customer. Sex workers were concerned about the risk to clients and had even told the police officers in the red-light district to inform their customers about the risks of not using condoms.[62]

Among women selling sex in Norway, there was a long tradition of using condoms at work. HIV/AIDS probably made it easier for sex workers to insist on using condoms.[63] Condom use was not only a pre-emptive measure to protect oneself from sexually transmitted infections, but also a way to protect 'the self'.[64] The condom was a piece of 'professional protective equipment' that served as a barrier between the body, which was her working tool, and her identity.[65] 'Nobody wants to contract sexually transmitted infections or get pregnant', a former sex worker and activist said. 'The condom was a protection against intimacy. It protected against semen. You didn't kiss the client or make out with him. You didn't want his semen inside of you. That was too intimate. In a way that was on your inside. It was a way to survive, to protect oneself.'[66] Another sex worker referred to the condom as an 'iron wall'.[67] A third described a situation where the condom broke and the customer came inside her: 'I panicked. I rinsed myself over and over again. I felt so dirty, but not because I was afraid of diseases or anything.'[68]

As sex workers became even more visible in Norwegian HIV/AIDS discourse in the later 1980s, this led to a more nuanced understanding among health authorities and social workers of the diversity of sex workers, their needs, and the situations and places in which the sale of sex took place. Officials increasingly acknowledged that sex was not only sold on the street but also in bars, hotel rooms, and through personal ads. Authorities and outreach services understood that the other part of the transaction, the client, must also be addressed. Therefore, the Pro Centre started a project dedicated to reaching out to clients, called the K-project.[69] Two social workers from the centre worked from a caravan in the red-light district of Oslo, from where they could make contact with customers either in person or through a new dedicated telephone hotline.

Officials also began to acknowledge that sex workers were a more heterogeneous group than previously thought, and that risk groups could not be neatly separated; some people used drugs, some were men, and some were even young boys.[70] These groups had different needs. In the first half of the 1980s, Uteseksjonen, a field service for drug users in Oslo, documented that boys were selling sex, often to men with whom they lived, and their lives were marked by violence, drug use, and shame.[71] At the beginning of the 1990s, the Pro Centre, in collaboration with the Gay Health Committee, started a project to find out more about this 'boy prostitution'.[72] The explicit aim of the project was not to 'eliminate prostitution as a phenomenon' or to 'rehabilitate boys who prostitute themselves', but to 'facilitate HIV prevention in these groups'. The outreach service approached this issue as 'a sexual relationship between two men involving a transaction' and focused on the exchange of sex or company for material goods such as money, housing, or clothing.

Instead of talking about 'prostitutes', the term 'boys/men who have experience of prostitution' was suggested in order to 'avoid further stigmatisation of persons in a stigmatised and taboo group'.[73]

While women usually worked in designated arenas, the project found that boys were more likely to work in crowded arenas like swimming pools, parks, and shopping malls, or through contact ads. Many were reported as having begun selling sex before the age of twelve and although money was given as a common motive, many were also said to have described excitement or sexual satisfaction.[74] The relationships between boys and 'customers' were also found to differ from those between female sex workers and their customers. Instead of money, gifts or services were often used as payment. Some boys described their relations with older men as providing warmth and care, or access to a secure grown-up. Many knew little about HIV prevention, such as the importance of combining water-based lube with condoms, and they often found themselves in vulnerable situations, unable to demand the use of a condom.[75] Some customers practised 'sero-sorting practices', meaning that they tried to identify who might be HIV-positive. The findings from the K-project and the 'boy prostitution' project led to a much deeper understanding of the complexities surrounding sex work. No single approach would suffice. Interventions had to be stratified and adjusted to account for gender and age, class and space.

Harm reduction policies: empowering sex workers

Having factual knowledge about HIV/AIDS and transmission mechanisms was one thing, but changing people's behaviour required more direct measures and personalised advice.[76] The official body overseeing Norwegian drug policy called for more individualised and low-threshold treatment, less bureaucratic services, and proper housing.[77] Some people had stopped selling sex due to the epidemic, but for others it had worsened the situation, especially for people using drugs.[78] Many had applied for rehabilitation services, but waiting lists were long. Harm-reducing measures such as the provision of clean syringes, training on syringe cleaning and hygienic preventive measures, as well as education work for pharmacists had to be intensified.

As in other countries, the HIV/AIDS epidemic led the Norwegian authorities to introduce harm-reduction approaches that sometimes considered those at risk as experts.[79] This started with drug users but continued with sex workers. Anne-Lise Middelthon recalled that when she started working for the Directorate of Health, which at that point had put together a team dedicated to HIV/AIDS, they realised that they knew too little about what was going on in situations where HIV transmission was a risk.[80] The authorities knew little about how people injected drugs or sold sex, and first-hand information and experience were needed. One way to get such information was to talk to the people involved. Officials in the AIDS team brought 'a bucket of syringes' to the municipal field service for drug users in Oslo, so that drug users could show them how they prepared and injected drugs. 'Then they showed us precisely what they were doing', Middelthon explained. 'Many of them aspirated the syringe and carefully examined the result.'[81]

At that time, a prevailing attitude among public health officials, substantiated by some anthropologists, was that sharing needles was a standard practice with great cultural significance among drug users.[82] From the authorities' point of view, this was seen as particularly dangerous since it would propagate the epidemic. However, when the AIDS team talked to people who used drugs, they found that people were already taking precautions to protect their health. These practices predated the epidemic. The syringe was rinsed before being passed on to others. If the whole dose was prepared at once, the second half would be aspirated after the first person had finished and rinsed out the syringe. Moreover, there was a hierarchy of who used the syringe first. The hierarchy sometimes reflected gendered power dynamics, such as a man injecting before a woman. However, it could also involve protective practices, with someone going last if they had just come down with the flu.[83] This practice was also maintained in the HIV/AIDS era, so that a person who had tested positive would receive the syringe towards the end to prevent the spread of the virus. According to Middelthon, many drug users spoke openly about their HIV status and their need to be the last person to use a shared syringe.[84]

Harm reduction policies were aimed at distributing syringes.[85] Throughout the epidemic, syringes were sold in pharmacies, and in 1988 free syringe distribution began in Oslo on a dedicated bus,

Sprøytebussen. This is an example of how HIV/AIDS prevention work in Norway crossed borders, with prevention among drug users and sex workers seen in relation to each other. Once more, working with the groups in question made social workers and authorities realise how heterogeneous they were. Kirsten Frigstad, one of the founders of the Pro Centre, was involved in this project and remembers how people from very different parts of society came to collect user equipment anonymously: 'They drove by with their BMWs and picked up syringes.'[86]

Eventually, many of the authorities' strategies for drug users were extended to sex workers, including the involvement of sex workers themselves in preventive work. They were inspired by leading sex workers' rights organisations in the USA, such as Coyote, which had established links between public health agencies and sex workers. There, HIV/AIDS had led to increased policing of sex workers and legal interventions such as mandatory testing. Coyote responded to this by working to reduce stigma and increase acceptance of prostitution as work, and began its own preventive efforts. In 1987, the California Prostitutes' Education Program, run by Coyote, began educating street sex workers about safer sex practices and intravenous hygiene.[87] Current and former sex workers provided educational materials and hosted information meetings and safe sex workshops. They went out to the streets to talk to women and men who sold sex about safer sex practices and provided condoms, bleach bottles, and spermicides. The programme also developed educational materials in versions adapted to different levels of education and literacy and using the vernacular of the trade, for instance, 'blow job' instead of 'fellatio' or 'oral sex'; 'domination' instead of 'S/M; and 'golden showers' rather than 'water sports'.[88]

The AIDS team in Norway was inspired by the Coyote project. They used the Coyote manual and visited them in San Francisco. Many sex workers had developed a technique of keeping the condom in the mouth before performing oral sex, then putting it on the penis without the customer noticing. The AIDS team saw sex workers train each other in this technique.[89] In 1987, one of the sex workers from San Francisco was invited to Norway to inspire similar work there.[90] However, to include sex workers directly in official preventive work was controversial among politicians and authorities, social workers, and the police. The planned meeting for social workers and sex workers to receive training in this technique and other preventive work took place, but sex workers were not mobilised to attend – although one former sex worker activist later said that this technique was already well-known among sex workers in Norway at the time, so it might not have made much difference.[91]

These initiatives faced additional problems. On behalf of the Directorate of Health, the Pro Centre recruited women to a peer education and prevention programme. But it was quickly realised that those women who were recruited who were *former* sex workers would not gain the necessary respect of those still involved in sex work. Ultimately, the authorities managed to find two women selling sex to deliver outreach work, and they were hired for ten hours per week. Anne-Lise Middelthon and Jo Kittelsen, who also worked for the AIDS team, recalled that for many people in different positions – from sex workers and social workers to the police and government officials – the roles of sex worker and employee just did not fit together.[92] The ultimate goal of politicians and those working with sex workers was to get them out of prostitution,[93] and employing sex workers was seen as an indirect legitimisation of sex work that contradicted this goal. Furthermore, would women be able to separate sex work from peer work? In the end, would the government pay women for selling sex? This kind of criticism demonstrated persistently stereotyped views of sex workers as unreliable and unable to distinguish between different roles. It also testifies to a stereotypical view of the 'sex worker' as an all-consuming identity, excluding other roles such as girlfriend, mother – or health worker. The AIDS team in the Directorate of Health saw this differently. Sex workers were appreciated for their proactive stance in reducing the risk of HIV transmission by the consistent use of condoms. They were even appreciated for providing public services by offering safer-sex education to colleagues and clients.

The two sex workers provided information about HIV/AIDS and distributed condoms and lubricant. Every day after work, they wrote detailed reports about their observations and experiences. In the beginning they had felt 'very insecure and afraid of being rejected by the prostitutes'.[94] But they quickly realised that their services were appreciated. They usually started the conversation by saying: 'Do you have time to talk to us for a bit? This is no harangue, we are not here to salvage you.'⁹⁵ One of the activists recalled that sex workers were particularly happy to receive free condoms. 'We had walked the same streets and we had worked in the same massage institutes. They knew who we were ... We knew all the prostitutes, where they tried to hide.'⁹⁶ As previously explained, the use of condoms was common, but many were not aware of the importance of using lubricants. These activist-employees also answered questions from sex workers about risks of infection and how to protect oneself: '[She] needs V and G [wet wipes and lube], gets inf. and stp. [information and vagitories]. When we mention N-9 [nonoxynol-9] in stp. and explain that it also kills HIV, she tells us that she is HIV-positive and asks if it will protect her boyfriend against HIV too. We tell her to use both.'⁹⁷ The women also brought something that was not directly related to reducing the risk of HIV: wet wipes. This was not part of a planned strategy, but many appreciated it. It was a sign that the authorities not only cared about risk reduction but cared about the women themselves, as people.⁹⁸

The Directorate of Health's programme on HIV/AIDS from 1988 emphasised that it was those who sold sex who should be made aware of the risk posed by the customer (see Figures 1.4 and 1.5).⁹⁹ Sex workers were no longer only 'vessels of infection', but were also approached as individuals with their own health risks and needs.

Conclusion: the politics of legitimation

Epidemics, and anxieties about venereal disease, have often activated dilemmas in governmental policy over individual rights and the need to protect society. Minorities and stigmatised groups have frequently been singled out. The arrival of HIV/AIDS, soon after a period of gender and sexual liberation, could have been exploited to enforce a backlash, and some have argued that this was the case, particularly in the early 1980s.¹⁰⁰ Norway was characterised by a high level of public trust in the health system and political systems, and a low level of distance between authorities and affected communities. This allowed for many official and unofficial networks and channels to hammer out and coordinate responses to HIV/AIDS. Empowering sexual minorities and reducing stigma and discrimination were objectives that fit well with governmental public

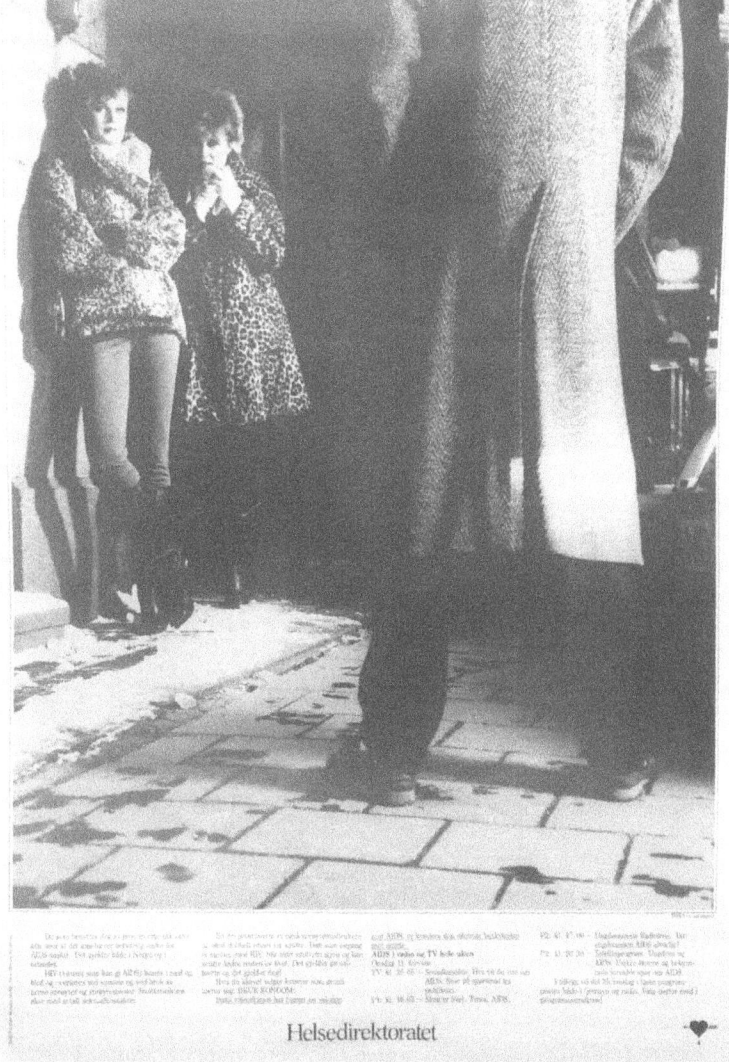

Figure 1.4 AIDS prevention poster, the Directorate of Health, 1987. 'You can buy AIDS'. The AIDS team commissioned an advertisement bureau to create posters for the campaign. This poster was never printed because the AIDS team was careful not to reproduce stereotypical and misogynistic depictions of sex workers, as Anne-Lise Middelthon said in an interview. (Copyright: ScanPartner/Anneks RRA6/Helsedirektoratet)

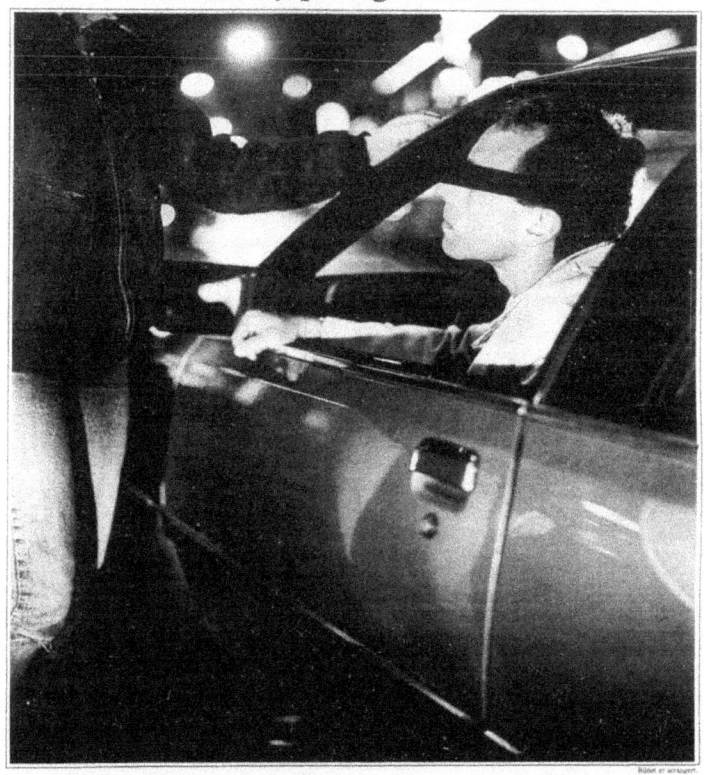

Figure 1.5 AIDS prevention poster, the Directorate of Health, 1987. 'You can buy AIDS'. Poster reprinted in several newspapers, aimed at customers. The text of the poster stated: 'Until the scientific community finds a vaccine against AIDS, the best protection is a condom'.
(Copyright: ScanPartner/Anneks RRA6/Helsedirektoratet)

health policy to participate in the fight against the oppression of sexual minorities. For this reason, it was relatively uncontroversial to include lesbian and gay activists in governmental HIV/AIDS work. From the beginning of the epidemic, lesbian and gay health workers played an important role in mediating between the state and those affected in their dual role as caregivers and members of the lesbian and gay community.[101]

For sex workers, however, the situation was different, especially at the beginning of the epidemic. Prostitution was an unwanted societal phenomenon, and policy goals focused on getting sex workers out of prostitution. In the second half of the 1980s, it was realised that sex workers were not the vectors of infection originally feared, and that they were a diverse group with differing needs. Most importantly, sex workers were increasingly seen as being at risk themselves, exposed to a number of health risks, including the effects of stigma and HIV/AIDS, rather than primarily a risk to others. Epidemiological work focused on identifying practices that could protect them. Although sex workers were stereotyped in the press and public health research, government policy began to support harm-reduction approaches. From the beginning, official prevention work with gay men was based on collaboration with activists, voluntary action, harm reduction, and empowering at-risk groups through a destigmatising approach. The same principles were eventually applied in official approaches to sex workers and their customers.

Sex worker activists played a similar role to lesbian and gay activists. They drew on embodied knowledge from their own lives and realities when providing information, educating peers about safer sex techniques, and distributing condoms and lubricant. However, even though sex workers were increasingly included in official preventive work, they never gained the expert status that the lesbian and gay community did.[102] One important reason was that sex workers had to challenge the hegemonic notion of sex work as a social problem: the materialisation of violence against women, commodification of the human body, and capitalist power structures. Another factor was that Norwegian sex workers lacked a platform from which to organise and stand up for their own rights.

HIV/AIDS changed this situation to some extent. The epidemic paved the way for new approaches to sex work in the public health sector and introduced harm-reduction policies for sex workers. More importantly, the epidemic spurred early sex work activism, made sex workers more vocal about their needs, and increasingly involved sex workers in governmental preventive work, as was also the case in other countries and contexts such as Germany and New Zealand.[103] Although sex workers still struggle to have their voices heard, the impact was long-lasting. In November 1990, the same sex and outreach workers who had been working on behalf of the government, together with Kirsten Frigstad from the Pro Centre, founded the first Norwegian activist organisation for sex workers, the 'Sex workers interest organisation in Norway' (PION).[104] PION still campaigns for the rights of sex workers today and opposes the criminalisation of sex work. This chapter of Norwegian HIV/AIDS history holds up alternatives to the use of legislative measures to combat an epidemic, based on engaging and collaborating with affected communities and activists through a non-stigmatising approach.

Acknowledgements

Ketil Slagstad and Anne Kveim Lie jointly planned the research project of which this chapter is part. Ketil Slagstad collected the archival material, conducted the oral history interviews, and wrote the first draft of the chapter. Both authors contributed to the analysis and co-wrote the final version of the chapter. Ketil Slagstad is grateful to the Science Studies Colloquium at the University of Oslo for providing a generous grant that made the project possible. Both authors are also immensely grateful to the interviewees who shared their stories with us, not least the former sex worker activists. A special thank you to Anne-Lise Middelthon, who opened her private archive and was available for valuable conversations. The authors also want to thank the staff at the Pro Centre and Helseutvalget for making their archives available, and the staff at the National Archives of Norway and Skeivt Arkiv for helping in the location of relevant material. Finally, the authors would like to express their gratitude to the editors of this volume, Janet Weston and

Hannah J. Elizabeth, whose comments and suggestions have greatly improved the chapter. The research for this chapter was funded by the Norwegian Research Council, grant number 283370, and the affiliated research project 'Biomedicalization from the Inside Out'.

Notes

1 Merill Singer, 'The politics of AIDS', *Social Science and Medicine*, 38:10 (1994), 1321–4.
2 The reader will notice that we are inconsistent in our terminology. We use 'prostitution', 'sex work', 'sex workers', and 'people selling sex'. We recognise that the distinction between these terms often has a political dimension and agree with Elizabeth Bernstein that 'sex work' is a broader, less stigmatising, and more neutral term. It is also the one preferred by sex worker activists and organisations, including the sex workers' interest organisation in Norway (PION). We have tried to stay as close to the primary sources as possible, using historically accurate terms. Some terms like 'prostitutes' [*prostituerte*] or 'hookers' [*horer*] have a pejorative and misogynist meaning, and we only use these when it is important to the historical analysis. To improve readability, we sometimes omit quotation marks when using these terms. Elizabeth Bernstein, *Temporarily yours: intimacy, authenticity, and the commerce of sex* (Chicago, IL: University of Chicago Press, 2007), pp. 17–18. All translations from Norwegian to English are ours.
3 But see Ketil Slagstad, 'The pasts, presents and futures of AIDS, Norway (1983–1996)', *Social History of Medicine*, 34.2 (2020), 417–44; Ketil Slagstad, 'The amphibious nature of AIDS activism: medical professionals and gay and lesbian communities in Norway, 1975–1987', *Medical History*, 64.3 (2020), 401–35.
4 May-Len Skilbrei, 'The development of Norwegian prostitution policies: a marriage of convenience between pragmatism and principles', *Sexuality Research and Social Policy*, 9.3 (2012), 244–57.
5 Liv Finstad, Lita Fougner, and Vivi-Lill Holter, *Prostitusjon i Oslo* (Oslo: Pax, 1982), p. 7.
6 Annika Snare and Cecilie Høigård, 'Noen trekk ved nordisk kvinnekriminologi', in *Kvinners skyld: en nordisk antologi i kriminologi*, ed. by Annika Snare and Cecilie Høigård (Oslo: Institutt for kriminologi og strafferett, Universitetet i Oslo, 1988), pp. 7–18.
7 See, for instance, the debate about this campaign in the radical feminists' own publication: 'Var «horekundeaksjonen» aksjonen forfeilet...?', *Kvinnefront*, 4 (1981), pp. 24–6. The left-wing newspaper

52   Histories of HIV/AIDS in Western Europe

   Klassekampen published a full-page story on its front page about the campaign, with the title 'Whoremongers in Oslo hunted down', depicturing feminists painting the cars of men who sought to buy sex; 'Horekunder jages i Oslo', *Klassekampen*, 11 April 1981, front page.
8 Skilbrei, 'The development of Norwegian prostitution policies'.
9 *Ibid.*
10 Finstad, Fougner, and Holter, *Prostitusjon i Oslo*, p. 7.
11 Pro Centre archive, Oslo (hereafter PCA), Vivi-Lill Holter, and Lita Fougner, 'Informasjonsprosjekt om prostitusjon 1. april–1. desember 1983'; PCA, Vivi-Lill Holter, 'Informasjonsprosjekt om prostitusjon, del II, 5. februar – 24. september 1984'.
12 Since January 2009 it has been illegal to buy sexual services in Norway.
13 For the moral fundament of the changes, see Svein Atle Skålevåg, 'Kjønnsforbrytelser. Sedelighet, seksualitet og strafferett 1880–1930', *Tidsskrift for kjønnsforskning*, 33.1–2 (2009), 7–25. Since then, the pimp paragraph has been changed several times.
14 The National Archives of Norway, Oslo (hereafter NAN), S-3454 Sosialdepartementet, Sosialavdelingen, 2, D, box 1654, folder 1, Prostitusjon, working paper by the Ministry of Justice, 'Kriminalisering av prostituertes kunder', December 1982.
15 Anne Stine Barli, Marina Berg, Bente Stoltz Berggrav, Kirsten Frigstad, Liv Jessen, Gunnar Nodland, Arne Randers-Pehrson, Mai Lisbeth Thoresen, and Mildrid Valvik, *Rapport fra akutthjemmet 1985*. PCA, Oslo Kommunes prostitusjonsprosjekt (Oslo: Rehabiliteringskontorets Akutthjem, 1985), p. 2.
16 Anne-Lise Middelthon's private archive (hereafter ALMA), opening speech by Astrid Nøkleby Heiberg in *Prostitusjon. Sosialdepartementets dagskonferanse 15 september 1982* (Oslo: Sosialdepartementet, 1983), p. 4; ALMA, speech by Martha Seim Valeur, 'Oslo kommunes arbeid mot prostitusjon', *Prostitusjon. Sosialdepartementets dagskonferanse 15 september 1982* (Oslo: Sosialdepartementet, 1983), p. 39.
17 PCA, Oslo Kommunes prostitusjonsprosjekt, *Rapport fra akutthjemmet 1986* (Oslo: Rehabiliteringskontorets Akutthjem, 1986).
18 PCA, Kirsten Frigstad 'Fra prosjekt til faste tiltak? Oppsummering av hjelpetiltakene' in *Prostitusjon i Norge – oppsummering av forskning og tiltak. Hva gjør vi nå?*, report from a seminar, 9 December 1988, University of Oslo.
19 Barli et al. *Rapport fra akutthjemmet 1985*, p. 4.
20 *Ibid.*
21 *Ibid.*
22 See Anne Kveim Lie, 'A commentary', *On learning from history: truths and eternal truths* (Oslo: Norges Bank, 2013); for the UK situation,

see Matt Cook, 'AIDS, mass observation, and the fate of the permissive turn', *Journal of the History of Sexuality*, 26.2 (2017), 239.
23 Jeffrey Weeks, 'AIDS and the regulation of sexuality', in *AIDS and contemporary history*, ed. by Virginia Berridge and Philip Strong (Cambridge: Cambridge University Press, 2002), pp. 17–36.
24 In 1989, Jeffrey Weeks argued that there had been three phases in the social response to the AIDS epidemic: 'the dawning crisis' (1981–2), 'moral panic' (1982–5), and 'crisis management' (1985–). Jeffrey Weeks, 'AIDS: the intellectual agenda', in *AIDS: social representation and social practices*, ed. by Peter Aggleton, Graham Hart, and Peter Davies (New York: The Falmer Press, 1989), pp. 1–20.
25 Paul Farmer, *AIDS and accusation: Haiti and the geography of blame* (Berkeley, CA: University of California Press, 2006).
26 Claude Quétel, *History of syphilis* (Cambridge: Polity Press, 1990), p. 16.
27 NAN, Pa-1216 Det Norske Forbundet av 1948, Db, box 7, AIDS, circular by the Ministry of Social Affairs, the Director General of Health to Norwegian hospitals, 'Rundskriv nr. 1. Ervervet immunsvikt syndrom (AIDS)', April 1983.
28 *Ibid.*
29 See Slagstad, 'The amphibious nature of AIDS activism'.
30 Carol Harris, Catherine Butkus Small, Robert S. Klein, Gerald H. Friedland, Bernice Moll, Eugene Emeson, Ilya Spigland, and Neal H. Steigbigel, 'Immunodeficiency in female sexual partners of men with the acquired immunodeficiency syndrome', *New England Journal of Medicine*, 308.20 (1983), 1181–4.
31 See, for instance, Robert R. Redfield, Phillip D. Markham, Syed Zaki Salahuddin, Craig D. Wright, M. G. Sarngadharan, and Robert C. Gallo, 'Heterosexually acquired HTLV-III/LAV disease (AIDS-related complex and AIDS): epidemiologic evidence for female-to-male transmission', *Journal of the American Medical Association*, 254.15 (1985), 2094–6; Randolph F. Wykoff, 'Female-to-male transmission of HTLV-III', *Journal of the American Medical Association*, 255.13 (1986), 1704–5; Robert R. Redfield, Craig D. Wright, Phillip D. Markham, Syed Zaki Salahuddin, M. G. Sarngadharan, and Robert C. Gallo, 'Female-to-male transmission of HTLV-III-reply', *Journal of the American Medical Association*, 255.13 (1986), 1705–6.
32 Paula A. Treichler, *How to have theory in an epidemic: cultural chronicles of AIDS* (Durham, NC: Duke University Press, 1999), pp. 18, 56–7.
33 Oslo City Archives, Oslo (hereafter OCA), Helserådet, box 52, AIDS, 'Helsedirektørens kontrollprogram for AIDS-sykdommen', 2 July 1985.

34 For a useful discussion of two ways of positioning vulnerable and minority groups as 'at risk' to others and 'at risk' personally, see Janet Weston, 'Sites of sickness, sites of rights? HIV/AIDS and the limits of human rights in British prisons', *Cultural and Social History*, 16.2 (2019), 225–40.
35 OCA, Helserådet, box 51, AIDS, letter from Thor Gundersen to Stadsfysikus Fredrik Mellbye, 3 September 1985.
36 *Ibid.*
37 Redfield et al., 'Heterosexually acquired HTLV-III/LAV disease'.
38 The National Library of Norway (hereafter NLN), 'Helsedirektørens tiltaksplan for bekjempelse av HIV-infeksjonen', AIDS-skriv nr. 17 (Oslo: Helsedirektoratet, 1986), pp. 13, 18.
39 NAN, Pa-1216 Det Norske Forbundet av 1948, Db, box 2, Sosialministerens referansegruppe, 'AIDS: Forebygging og kontroll av HIV-infeksjoner. Forslag til intensivert målrettet smitteoppsporing og konkrete tiltak og virkemidler mot smittemottakere og smittekilder', AIDS-skriv nr. 21 (Oslo: Helsedirektoratet, 1 March 1987).
40 ALMA, *AIDS: Handlingsprogram for skolerings- og opplysningsarbeid om HIV/AIDS* (Oslo: Helsedirektoratet, 1 September 1988), p. 10.
41 *Ibid.*, p. 9.
42 NAN, 'AIDS: Forebygging og kontroll av HIV-infeksjoner', p. 15.
43 ALMA, *AIDS: Handlingsprogram for skolerings- og opplysningsarbeid om HIV/AIDS*, p. 10.
44 Stig Frøland, *AIDS – en utfordring til oss alle* (Oslo: Gyldendal, 1986), p. 169.
45 Anne Sissel Skånvik and Karin Bøhm-Pedersen, 'AIDS blant Oslo-horer', *Dagbladet*, 20 June 1985, p. 10.
46 Janice Delaney, Mary Jane Lupton, and Emily Toth, *The curse: a cultural history of menstruation* (Champaign: University of Illinois Press, 1988).
47 Arvid Bryne, 'Jeg er en levende dødsmaskin', *Dagbladet*, 6 August 1985, p. 9.
48 See, for instance, Allan M. Brandt, *No magic bullet: a social history of venereal disease in the United States since 1880* (New York: Oxford University Press, 1985); Judith R. Walkowitz, *Prostitution and Victorian society: women, class, and the state* (Cambridge: Cambridge University Press, 1980).
49 Mary Spongberg, *Feminizing venereal disease: the body of the prostitute in nineteenth century medical discourse* (Basingstoke: Macmillan, 1997).
50 The concept of a 'virus' had a very different meaning at that time.
51 Walkowitz, *Prostitution and Victorian society*.

52 Priscilla Alexander, *Prostitutes prevent AIDS: a manual for health educators* (San Francisco, CA: California Prostitutes Education Project [CAL-PEP], 1988).
53 See also Treichler, *How to have theory in an epidemic*, pp. 61–2.
54 See, for instance, Karin Bøhm-Pedersen, 'Kan ikke sperre AIDS-hore inne' ['Cannot lock up AIDS hookers'], *Dagbladet*, 1 July 1985, p. 9; Jorunn Stølan og Frode Holst, 'Uthengt som AIDS-hore' ['Mocked as AIDS hooker'], *VG*, 16 May 1987, p. 17; 'Kjøpte sex av AIDS-hore' ['Bought sex from AIDS hooker'], *VG*, 20 May 1988, front page. We agree with Skilbrei that even if the Norwegian word 'hore' shares the etymology of the English word 'whore', semantically it is closer to 'hooker'; see Skilbrei, 'The development of Norwegian prostitution policies'.
55 Anne Sissel Skånvik, 'AIDS skremmer ikke horekunder' ['AIDS does not scare away hooker customers'], *Dagbladet*, 21 June 1985, p. 7.
56 Susan Sontag, *AIDS and its metaphors* (New York: Farrar, Straus and Giroux, 1989), p. 11.
57 'Siv (30) – hore med AIDS' ['Siv (30) – hooker with AIDS'], *Dagbladet*, 29 June 1985, pp. 7–9.
58 What was lost in the media reporting was the widespread use of condoms by sex workers in Norway. See the next section.
59 PCA, Anne Eskild, Ingela Kvalem, and Jon Martin Sundet, 'Use of condoms by prostitutes', Norwegian Institute of Public Health. Undated.
60 PCA, Anne Eskild, *Helsetilstand og helsetjenestebruk i et utvalg prostituerte kvinner i Oslo: En intervjuundersøkelse* (Oslo: Statens institutt for folkehelse, 1988).
61 Ibid.
62 PCA, Oslo politikammer, Prostitusjon- og hallikspanegruppen, Orientering, 26 April 1990.
63 Ibid.
64 Anne-Lise Middelthon, 'De farlige andre: Om anti-struktur og metaforiserings- og metonymiseringsprosesser i hiv-epidemien' (master's thesis, University of Oslo, 1992), pp. 44–7.
65 We are indebted to Anne-Lise Middelthon for this term. See also Sophie Day, 'Prostitute women and AIDS: anthropology', *AIDS*, 2.6 (1988), 421–8.
66 Sex worker activist in interview with Ketil Slagstad, Oslo, 19 August 2019. The interviewee wished to remain anonymous.
67 Middelthon, 'De farlige andre', p. 47.
68 Ibid.
69 'K' for 'kunde', the Norwegian word for customer.

70 ALMA, *AIDS: Handlingsprogram for skolerings- og opplysningsarbeid om HIV/AIDS*, p. 14.
71 Skeivt arkiv, Bergen (hereafter SA), A-0078 Helseutvalget, Da, box 31, folder 8, 'Prosjekt for å nå unge gutter som prostituerer seg for å muliggjøre forebyggende HIV-arbeid. Prosjektbeskrivelse', 8 October 1990.
72 SA, A-0078 Helseutvalget, Da, box 31, folder 8, Asbjørn Solevåg, 'Handlingsplan for Pro-senterets gutteprosjekt', 10 April 1991.
73 *Ibid*. As this suggests, boys were not conceputalised as children experiencing abuse, but as boys engaging in sex work.
74 PCA, Årsrapport 1991 Pro-senterets gutteprosjekt, p. 9.
75 *Ibid.*, p. 16.
76 ALMA, *AIDS: Handlingsprogram for skolerings- og opplysningsarbeid om HIV/AIDS*, p. 11.
77 NAN, S-3454 – Sosialdepartementet, Alminnelig avdeling/ Sosialavdelingen, 2, D, box 149, Permanente kommisjoner, nemder og råd, Sentralrådet for narkotikaproblemer 1987–1990, 'Behov for strakstiltak for behandling av stoffmisbrukere', 22 September 1987.
78 PCA, *Rapport fra akutthjemmet 1986* p. 4.
79 See, for instance, Ine Vanwesenbeeck and Ron de Graaf, 'Sex work and HIV in the Netherlands: policy, research and prevention', in *The Dutch response to HIV: pragmatism and consensus*, ed. by Theo Sandfort (London: UCL Press, 1998), pp. 86–106.
80 The following section is based on an interview of Anne-Lise Middelthon by Ketil Slagstad, Oslo, 23 January 2019.
81 Middelthon interview, 23 January 2019.
82 Middelthon, 'De farlige andre', pp. 48–50; Nina Glick Schiller, 'What's wrong with this picture? The hegemonic construction of culture in AIDS research in the United States', *Medical Anthropology Quarterly*, 6 (1992), 237–54.
83 ALMA, 'Intervju med 4 erfarne sprøytebrukere som kom til Uteseksjonen 13.10.1987'. Interviews with four experienced injecting drug users, two women and two men, who came to Uteseksjonen [The Outreach Service] on 13 October 1987. The interviews were conducted by Anne-Lise Middelthon, Jo Kittelsen, and Mona Duckert in the waiting area of Uteseksjonen.
84 Middelthon interview, 23 January 2019.
85 ALMA, *Gateprostitusjon i Bergen. Prosjektrapport august 1984 – juli 1986* (Bergen: Kommunalavdeling helse og sosiale tjenester, 1988), pp. 15–16.

86 Kirsten Frigstad in interview with Ketil Slagstad, Oslo, 19 March 2019. Frigstad was the director of the Pro Centre throughout the 1980s.
87 Valerie Jenness, 'From sex as sin to sex as work: COYOTE and the reorganization of prostitution as a social problem', *Social Problems*, 37.3 (1990), 403–20.
88 Alexander, *Prostitutes prevent AIDS*, p. 20.
89 Nancy Shaw and Lyn Paleo, 'Women and AIDS', in *What to do about AIDS: physicians and mental health professionals discuss the issues*, ed. by Leon McKusick (Berkeley, CA: University of California Press, 1986), pp. 142–54.
90 Anonymous sex worker activist interview with Ketil Slagstad, 19 August 2019.
91 Middelthon interview, 23 January 2019; Jo Kittelsen in interview with Ketil Slagstad, Oslo, 14 March 2019.
92 Middelthon interview, 23 January 2019; Kittelsen interview, 14 March 2019.
93 As reflected in the title of a book written by the leaders of the Pro Centre, *The girls: out of prostitution*; Liv Jessen and Kirsten Frigstad, *Jentene – ut av prostitusjonen* (Oslo: J.W. Cappelen forlag, 1988).
94 ALMA, report to the AIDS team in the Directorate of Health, 10 January 1989. The two women wrote reports from their work that were handed over to the AIDS team at the Directorate of Health. One of them has approved the use of these reports in this chapter.
95 *Ibid.*
96 Anonymous sex worker activist interview with Ketil Slagstad, 19 August 2019.
97 ALMA, report to the Directorate of Health, 6 December 1989. Nonoxynol-9 was at that time believed to reduce the risk of HIV transmission.
98 Middelthon, 'De farlige andre', pp. 64–5; Middelthon interview, 23 January 2019.
99 ALMA, *AIDS: Handlingsprogram for skolerings- og opplysningsarbeid om HIV/AIDS*, p. 14.
100 Weeks, 'AIDS: the intellectual agenda'.
101 Slagstad, 'The amphibious nature'.
102 *Ibid.* For the US situation, see Steven Epstein, *Impure science: AIDS, activism, and the politics of knowledge* (Los Angeles, CA: University of California Press, 1996).

103 Cheryl Ware, 'Sex workers' responses to the HIV and AIDS epidemic in Aotearoa New Zealand', *Women's History Review*, 29.2 (2020), 289–307; Mareen Heying, 'The German prostitutes' movement: *Hurenbewegung*. From founding to law reform, 1980–2002', *Moving the Social*, 59 (2018), 24–45.

104 Frigstad interview, 19 March 2019; sex worker activist interview, 19 August 2019. PION was the abbreviation for Prostituertes interesseorganisasjon [The Organisation for Prostitutes], which later changed its name to 'The sex workers interest organisation in Norway'.

2

Drug criminalisation, the Catholic Church, and the 1988 founding of a Rome AIDS care centre

Brian DeGrazia

This chapter begins with the controversial 1988 founding of an AIDS care centre in Rome: the Villa Glori Casa famiglia per malati di AIDS, or simply the Casa famiglia. It examines the discussion that this centre sparked in the Italian media, and media depictions of HIV/AIDS in circulation more generally at the time in Italy, including the language surrounding HIV/AIDS in official governmental communications. These were, as I argue, highly stigmatising and positioned drug users as a threat to the safety of (upper- and middle-class, heterosexual) Italian families. Finally, it places these failings within the Italian response to HIV/AIDS in a global context, shaped by the American 'War on Drugs'.

The history of HIV/AIDS in Italy has remained largely understudied and merits particular attention because of the country's distinctive epidemiological and cultural profile. The predominance of intravenous drug use, in both epidemiological terms and in popular discourse about the epidemic, means that careful attention to Italy offers a different perspective from the better-known histories of HIV/AIDS in countries like the United States of America (USA) and the United Kingdom (UK), and their focus on gay men. Although concentrated on Italy, this chapter also situates itself in a necessarily international context, with politics on the global stage playing a significant role. The controversy that delayed the opening of the Casa famiglia coincided with the passing of stricter drug legislation in the USA, and the visit of Italian Socialist Party Secretary Bettino Craxi to New York and Washington, DC to discuss related matters. The confluence of these events and their conflation in government and media discourse alike led to the effective criminalisation of HIV/AIDS in Italy and a long-lasting stigmatisation of drug users in particular. Situated in Rome's affluent Parioli neighbourhood, Villa Glori was inaugurated on 18 May 1924 as the Park of Remembrance and was originally intended as a dedicatory space for Italians who had died in the First World War. The park later became a place to remember the fallen more broadly; its monuments commemorate military casualties that range from the nineteenth-century Risorgimento to the twenty-first century war in Iraq.[1] Five years after its inauguration, the park became home to its first healthcare-related facility, the Colonia Marchiafava, named for Italian physician and pathologist Ettore Marchiafava. From 1929, this colony hosted children of poor families with tuberculosis or other illnesses during summers. Its location was chosen quite deliberately; it was hoped that the fresh, clean air in this lush park atop a hill on the outskirts of the city of Rome would bring salubrious effects to the children spending summers there.[2]

The repurposing of these facilities into a home for people with HIV/AIDS (PWHA) was therefore not entirely foreign to their original purpose. The Roman city government approved 'the establishment of a residential community for citizens affected by AIDS at the Villa Glori complex' in early July 1988, leaving the management of the facility to the Catholic welfare organisation Caritas. The centre's first nine residents were expected to arrive in the autumn of that year and, unlike the seasonal nature of the original colony, to remain year-round.[3] The Casa famiglia was led by don Luigi di Liegro, the president of Caritas in Rome. Before heading Caritas, di Liegro had worked as a pastor in the city, and by the late 1980s had a reputation not only for spearheading a wide array of initiatives to help poorer and disenfranchised communities, but also for speaking out when necessary against politicians, clergy, and the citizens of the city in order to carry out his missions. Director Luigi Faccini, in his 1989 film about the Casa famiglia, anecdotally explained that 'a few days ago, a Roman taxi driver recognised [di Liegro] as the one who defends gypsies, and made him get out of the car'.[4] The controversy surrounding the Casa famiglia was therefore not di Liegro's first brush with opposition, but it landed him in the spotlight of the national news media for several months before the Casa famiglia finally opened in December.

The Casa famiglia sought to offer space to young people who were without a stable home, because their families either could not or refused to provide for them. The initiative focused specifically on those who were using or had used drugs, particularly heroin. This responded to the emerging epidemiological data in Italy, which indicated very high rates of HIV/AIDS among young people who used intravenous drugs. 'Drug addiction', according to a 1994 Italian medical textbook, 'is the most represented category' among those diagnosed with HIV or AIDS, with about 70 per cent of AIDS diagnoses and 63.7 per cent of new HIV diagnoses attributed to it.[5] The sharing of needles and syringes, then, appeared to be the principal mode of HIV transmission in Italy and, equally, a large number of intravenous drug users contracted HIV/AIDS. In Milan, the city worst affected by HIV/AIDS among drug users, the rate of infection within this group jumped from 5 to 50 per cent in just three years, peaking at 67 per cent in 1987. Similar figures were seen throughout the country, albeit with the north and urban centres most severely affected.[6]

The founding of the Casa famiglia in Rome was significant not only as one of the first events to drive a national conversation about HIV/AIDS in Italy, but also as a point of convergence of the two factors that rendered the Italian iteration of the epidemic unique: the role of intravenous drug use, and the role of the Church in delivering services.[7] As one private citizen remarked when voicing his resistance to the Casa famiglia, 'Initiatives like this [are] "American-style" initiatives to cover up the collapse of the public health system'.[8] In the face of a lack of public services and a largely phobic and intolerant reaction from private citizens, and despite some of the moral and ideological stances of the Church that seemingly prevented valuable engagement with the epidemic, Caritas stepped in. It provided through the Casa famiglia a stop-gap service for a small group of young people. As the next section shows, the reactions to this service as well as the service itself were revealing; they were indicative of broader concerns, and particularly a fear of social rather than biomedical contagion.

'Villa Glori cannot become a dealers' hideout': resistance to the Casa famiglia

There was a need for places where people with HIV/AIDS could access reliable medical advice, care, and treatment, given the deficiencies of both public and private healthcare concerning HIV/AIDS in Italy. A handful of high-profile Italian doctors were among the first to proclaim this need publicly and repeatedly. A television special entitled *AIDS: Between Science and Society* [*AIDS: Tra scienza e società*] aired on 13 December 1988 on Rai 1.[9] The programme was financed and produced by L'Associazione nazionale per la lotta contro l'Aids (Anlaids), an organisation founded in 1985 by a team of doctors, researchers, journalists, activists, and volunteers, which is still in operation today.[10] Nearly the whole programme was dedicated to interviews with two doctors, both vice presidents of Anlaids: Dr Mauro Moroni, a well-known infectious disease specialist at the Ospedale Luigi Sacco in Milan, and Dr Guido Rondanelli, clinical director at the specialised school for infectious diseases at the University of Pavia. Both of them, and Moroni in particular, emphasised the urgent need for volunteers to join the effort in responding to HIV/AIDS, as a supplement to government funding and medical research.

While Moroni and Rondanelli were calling for the intervention of activists and volunteers, Dr Fernando Aiuti publicly decried the lack of hospital space and medical staff for PWHA and connected this to the activities of Caritas at Villa Glori. Aiuti, director of the school of immunology at La Sapienza in Rome and an authority on HIV/AIDS in Italy from the outset of the epidemic, repeatedly stated that the epidemic had been underestimated by many, largely because he and other experts had been ignored. Interviewing Aiuti on the television programme *Viaggio intorno all'uomo*, which aired on Rai 3 on 28 October 1988, journalist Sergio Zavoli asked Aiuti about the situation in rather drastic and alarmist terms: 'Professor Aiuti, the day when the disease should become, so to speak, hospitalised, would that not mean the collapse of healthcare structures, which are already so deficient in our country?' Aiuti agreed.

> I think this day has already come. There will not be long to wait now, perhaps a few months, because unfortunately the sick are growing

in number and if measures are not taken to hospitalise these AIDS patients beyond infectious disease wards, but rather in internal medicine wards designated for the care of these patients, we will have to have recourse to other solutions.[11]

Aiuti concluded by acknowledging the presence of di Liegro of Caritas and the Casa famiglia as a fellow guest, and spoke supportively of di Liegro's work. He clarified here and later that services such as those provided by Caritas were valuable for those in reasonable health, but were no replacement for proper medical care where that was needed. Further explaining this issue two months later in a half-hour-long interview on Radio 1's *Sotto tiro* with Paolo Conti, Aiuti reaffirmed his support for Caritas, and the value of residential centres to compensate for the lack of hospital space, adding again that 'a residence does not substitute for a hospital. The hospital must be the primary objective, and thus I do not want, with the creation of many residences, for people to forget that the hospital is open day and night and does not discriminate against anyone'.[12]

Aiuti's support for the Caritas initiative no doubt constituted an important endorsement in what had already become a heated battle to open the Casa famiglia. His words of caution about the limits of non-medical residential facilities, as the opinion of a medical professional, also likely emboldened Parioli residents who presented a host of arguments against this centre in their neighbourhood.

Such dissent began to emerge in the pages of some of Italy's largest dailies and on television news broadcasts at the beginning of October 1988. One woman from the Parioli neighbourhood echoed one of Aiuti's suggestions to refurbish and bring back into use old, empty hospitals. 'There's a hospital that was built but never used at Grottarossa. Let them use that', she reportedly said.[13] Fausto Maria Puccini, another Parioli resident, expressed concerns about the standard of facilities at the Casa famiglia when interviewed for an early October article in *Corriere della Sera*: 'The residence is not in keeping with the health code, nor does it have the assistance necessary for AIDS patients, who should be spending their days in the hospital and not in a country villa. The bathroom is close to the kitchen; a group of people who saw it told us.'[14] Puccini, a local lawyer and businessman, became one of the most outspoken figures in opposition to the Caritas initiative. He also owned the

Grand Hotel Ritz Roma, just blocks from the entrance to Villa Glori, which would eventually host a gathering of local residents to discuss their concerns and organise a protest march through the park the following weekend.[15] Petitions had circulated to collect the signatures of those opposed to the Casa famiglia, which Puccini would eventually bring before the Tribunale Amministrativo Regionale in an effort to stop the Casa famiglia from opening.[16]

Dino Martirano's article in the *Corriere della Sera* quotes Puccini and other local residents without overt comment, but implicitly endorses their fears as valid. Indeed, the article begins with a discussion of fear of HIV/AIDS in general and of the Casa famiglia in particular.

> AIDS causes fear. It causes fear from watching informational spots on TV and reading the statistics of the victims published in the newspapers. But the disease of the century sows terror when it manifests itself in the public garden outside one's door, with the apparition of a centre, immersed in the greenery, for patients affected by the 'acquired immunodeficiency syndrome'.[17]

HIV/AIDS was characterised as always fear-inducing, but downright terrifying when it presented itself within a certain spatial proximity. Here, it became a 'seed' of terror, planted in the garden outside one's home. This seed, ironically, was itself a home. The article's introduction, along with its accompanying title and subtitles, incited alarmism based on proximity to HIV/AIDS, and although proximity to HIV/AIDS necessarily meant proximity to PWHA, those people were themselves elided here.

The article describes the idyllic beauty of the park and its use as a luscious outdoor sanctuary for dog owners, runners, and especially young families with children. The author included fragments of his conversations with some of these young couples and mothers, and the single photograph used to illustrate the article, as well as one of the quoted statements above it that the 'park will be abandoned by the children', emphasised the view that the park was properly a refuge for families and young children and that this was under threat. One of the young mothers explained more precisely what she and her neighbours feared with the imminent opening of the Casa famiglia. 'It's been a few days now that we have been discussing this affair and I can say that we are not against persons with AIDS, but rather seriously worried about what the opening of the centre will bring with it. I am talking about the sick who are addicts and the possibility that they bring along with them all the delinquency linked to the selling of drugs.' Another young couple suggested establishing the centre elsewhere, and reiterated these same fears, asking, 'Why here and not somewhere else? They could set up AIDS patients on the Cassia or in some country house.' The husband clarified that the 'problem is not AIDS patients, but the presence of others that they will provoke. And', he added, citing the political activity discussed at the end of this chapter, 'we do not believe at all in the measures that the state and the police announce in the fight against the sale of drugs'.[18]

This article opened by saying that AIDS caused fear, but these individuals were very forthcoming about the fact that it was not AIDS that scared them, but the people they associated with it. In their view, the residents of the Casa famiglia would bring with them a culture of drugs and delinquency. *This* was what sowed terror: drugs, and those who used and sold them. Martirano, in his conclusion to the article, also made this explicit.

> Thus, in a neighbourhood where the average level of education is certainly not stuck in the fifth grade, the frequenters of Villa Glori demonstrate that they know many things about AIDS and about the possibility of contracting the virus, which is only transmitted through blood and sexual relations. But the idea that persons infected with 'acquired immunodeficiency syndrome' could bring to the park all the contradictions that erupt on a daily basis in other parts of the city does not let them rest easy.

The contrast drawn here between the wealthy neighbourhood of Parioli with its well-educated residents and 'other parts of the city' heads off any criticisms of ignorant prejudice, and implies that the residents of Parioli are wise to fear drug users and dealers who might come to and contaminate their beloved park.

Neighbourhood residents expressed more concerns of this nature when they gathered two days later at Puccini's hotel. Puccini himself went so far as to call di Liegro a liar, stating that he 'lies when he says that there will be nine youngsters at the beginning and then twenty in all. They can grow to great numbers and they will wander freely in the park taken away from families. It's not true that it will just be a home. There will even be doctors.'[19] One concerned mother reportedly shouted, 'It's a bomb fused right before the children's eyes!'[20] 'Villa Glori cannot become a dealers' hideout', another exclaimed.[21] In a television broadcast rife with images of children and pushchairs in the park, this was repeated again in a plea from one interviewee to 'leave at least the public parks for the children, for the elderly, for the people'.[22] Notably, she used the word *gente* for people, which has connotations of the upper classes, rather than *popolo*, which is often associated with the middle and lower classes or the population as a whole. If other Parioli residents spoke about drug dealers and drug users in vague terms that presented them as a collective nebulous threat, this woman's call for the park to be kept for the 'people' categorically dehumanised them; Villa Glori should be reserved for 'people' only.

Drug sale and use were problems that, in the eyes of the inhabitants of the wealthy Parioli neighbourhood, belonged to the city's poorer areas. The opposition to the Casa famiglia at Villa Glori marked the third time in a year that di Liegro had met the vociferous and exclusionary objections of residents of neighbourhoods who did not want to accommodate unwelcome 'others'; the previous two incidents, however, had to do with the settlement of Rome's Roma population in the area around Termini Station and in the city's periphery.[23] A few Pariolini drew direct comparisons with these recent events, stating that 'People with AIDS are worse than gypsies, who at least don't have infectious diseases.'[24] Some took to ad hominem verbal insults of di Liegro. Even those who did not mention these disputes likely already knew who di Liegro was. The Pariolini who spoke out largely saw him not as a figure of charity and volunteer work, but as a driver of social contamination, bringing groups that were either socially or spatially marginalised into richer and more desirable neighbourhoods in the city centre, where they and their problems did not belong.

'Reprehensible are those who…': messages from medical authorities

To understand the atmosphere in which the Casa famiglia met with such adamant protest, it is worth looking at the messages emanating from the Italian Ministry of Health and its similarly insidious rhetoric. On the occasion of the first global World AIDS Day on 1 December 1988, Carlo Donat-Cattin, the Italian minister of health, mailed a letter about HIV/AIDS to all Italian families. In the second bullet point of six, Donat-Cattin dismissed a common metaphor for the epidemic, clarifying that 'AIDS is not the plague as described by Manzoni in *The betrothed*: it does not infect through the air, nor through contact with clothing, furniture, or people. No. The AIDS virus is transmitted only through blood and sexual secretions by an already-infected person to a non-infected person.'[25] From there, however, the letter traded scientific precision for pernicious ambiguities with moralising overtones.

'There exist at-risk categories', the letter continues, 'and behaviours: haemophiliacs, homosexuals, drug users, et cetera'. The naming of haemophiliacs first is curious; there was no information to pass on to haemophiliacs in terms of precautions that they could take, since their risks arose from iatrogenic error in the form of a lack of diligence and testing of donated blood. The case was different for (largely male) homosexuals and intravenous drug users, who, with proper information and resources, could have learned more about means of transmission, about riskier and safer behaviours, and lowered their chances of contracting the virus. Yet, this letter contained no information for them about how to reduce risks, and with its ill-placed 'et cetera' at the end of the sentence, it left readers uncertain and anxious as to who or what else might be 'at risk'. Without specifics or practical advice for those who could take preventive measures, the letter simply identified those who should be fearful – and potentially also feared.

This was not the only way in which the letter stoked stigmatisation. The bullet point concluded that 'since AIDS has been spreading, even families or communities who feel far away from the danger must not neglect to take some precautions'. This juxtaposition created a conceptual divide between those in the at-risk categories on one hand and 'families and communities' on the other. Non-heterosexuals and drug users often did find themselves ostracised from their families and other communities, as demonstrated by the hostility of the Parioli community towards the Villa Glori Casa famiglia. More dangerously, this division insinuated that those in 'at-risk' categories constituted a point of origin from which the disease would spread and threaten 'families and communities'.[26]

The family, as Donat-Cattin was keen to reiterate, constituted the central building block of Italian society. 'The Constitution of the Republic', he writes in the letter, 'recognises and safeguards the family. The family is normally the ideal place for an effective interpersonal equilibrium in the fight against AIDS.' The family could indeed become an important resource if it encouraged open and honest dialogue and provided support. In the context of this letter, however, such an assertion presented the family as a kind of bulwark against social and sexual delinquencies, undertaken by abnormal persons who lacked a sense of Christian morality. The third bullet point and the first half of the fourth are worth reproducing in their entirety.

> 3. The Ministry of Health must give instructions that are useful and as complete as possible to help understand and fight the disease, for those who adhere to a religious or lay morality, and for those who seek to avoid it. With the first group, the question is simpler. With the second it is more complex: campaigns of all kinds try to be persuasive about a perfect way to prevent the disease and, thus, to practise risky lifestyles. But this is not possible. Those who affirm, for example, the absolute safety of condoms, are proven wrong by almost all the experts. We have written: 'It is not entirely safe.' For now, the condom is the only barrier for dangerous sexual encounters, but a barrier with limits: this is the reason behind the absurdity of the idea that the condom permits any lifestyle, without risk.
>
> 4. For a healthy person, the first rule to which it is advisable to adhere is that of a normal existence with regard to romantic and sexual relationships. There are a host of health-related reasons to behave with balance, even if little weight is given to the moral ones. This rule, according to many doctors, is also valid for the seropositive. Jokes can be made about chastity. It is, however, indicated by the World Health Organization as the first choice for the comportment of the seropositive; for people who are not sick with AIDS, but who are carries of the virus, who, if they have a sense of responsibility, must act so as not to transmit the infection.[27]

With the use of the word 'normal', as Vittorio Agnoletto argues, 'all those who do not adhere to the wishes of the Ministry become "abnormal", and as such are candidates for contracting the virus'.[28] By dividing social and sexual practices along the lines of moral and immoral, normal and abnormal, those with HIV/AIDS can be held responsible and positioned as dangerous. Donat-Cattin may have attempted to distance HIV/AIDS from the plague and from Manzoni, but his moralising and sometimes threatening letter established logics of blame and hierarchies of people as either threatening or innocent that echo Manzoni's *History of the column of infamy* as well as *The betrothed*. 'From this moment', concludes Agnoletto, 'AIDS is no longer a disease but a fault, and the virus is the sign of the sin'.[29]

Those refusing the 'normal' life of the heterosexual couple would seem to pose the greatest moral and epidemiological threat to Italian society. Even more dangerous, however, are those who are not even mentioned in the development of this logic: intravenous drug users. Donat-Cattin does damage by sowing seeds of doubt about condom use, but arguably does even more harm by writing nothing at all about how the virus spreads among those who use intravenous drugs, and what precautions they might take. 'Drug users', according to the letter, do constitute a 'risk category', but there is apparently nothing to be done in relation to drug use to stop the virus from spreading and threatening the sacrosanct family unit. The drug user might be the most dangerous threat of all.

One of the Health Ministry's first television adverts about HIV/AIDS, aired in early 1990, propagated this logic in visual terms.[30] The advert begins with a stern voiceover stating that AIDS itself is not visible but 'is spreading'. Within the first few seconds, the advert temporarily overcomes this invisibility as the camera moves to show an overhead view of a series of compartments, which seem like a series of bathroom stalls, within some kind of large industrial complex. The two young men who step into the first compartment close the door behind them, presumably in an effort not to be seen and reflecting again the invisibility of the virus (were it not for the camera hovering above them).

The silhouette of the body of one of the men is outlined in neon purple, signifying the body of a seropositive person. This is reinforced by a stripe of the same colour that underlines the word 'AIDS' in the first image, as shown in Figure 2.1. Over the sound of a pulsating beep in the background akin to an electrocardiogram, the voiceover explains that 'AIDS cannot be seen, but it is growing. Because it is transmitted *not only* through infected blood… for example, using the same syringe'. At this moment, the second man

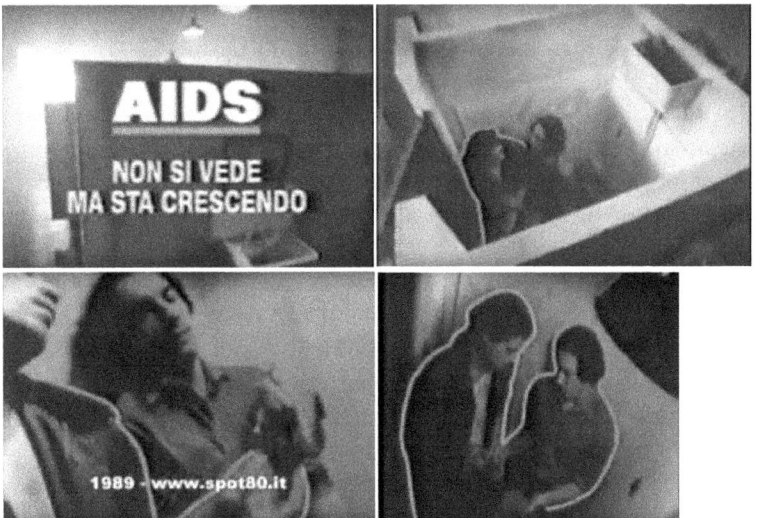

Figure 2.1 Stills from the beginning of 'AIDS: Non si vede ma sta crescendo', a television advert released by the Ministry of Health in 1990.

takes the syringe from the first and injects its contents into his arm; the purple outline expands to cover the second man as well, indicating transmission of the virus. The camera freezes on the couple as the second man injects – the only freeze-frame in the advert – and a long pause follows the word 'syringe'. This, the viewer is being told, is the most significant moment.

Figure 2.2 gives an indication of the rest of the advert. The second man then leaves the strange, dystopic space where he shared the syringe and moves into a much more recognisable social setting: a bar, full of people. His confused, vacant stare from earlier has transformed into a smile with this change of scenery. He sees people he knows and talks with them briefly before leaving the bar to head home with one of them, a young woman. A shot of the two of them in bed together shows the purple outline spreading around her as well, indicating that she has contracted the virus through unprotected sex with this man. The woman will eventually go on to sleep with one of her co-workers before he, dressed in suit and tie to indicate his high socio-economic status, enters the space of his own home – the space of the family, 'recognised and safeguarded' by the constitution – with the purple outline around him.

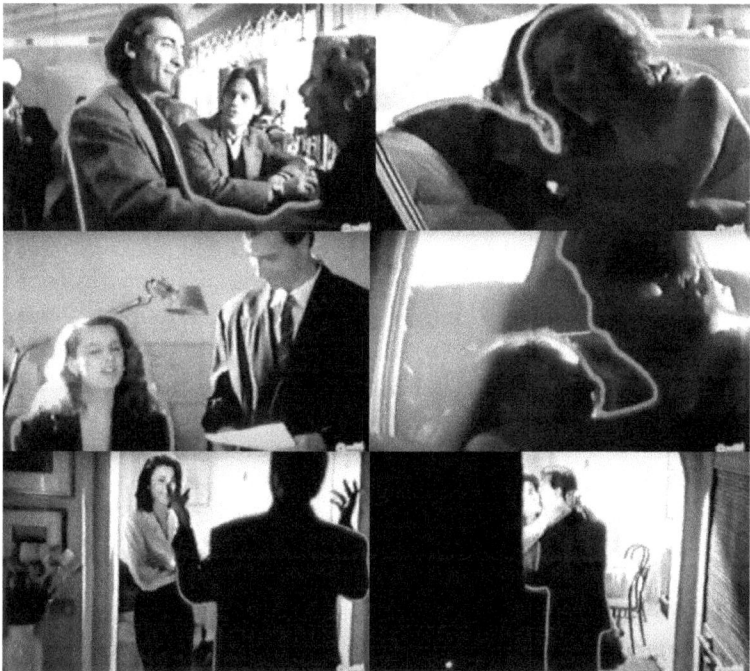

Figure 2.2 Stills from 'AIDS: Non si vede ma sta crescendo', a television advert released by the Ministry of Health in 1990.

He and his wife, unlike others in the advert, are entitled to privacy and this time the closing door shuts out the camera. In the narrative constructed by this advert, the virus has thus made its way from the strange, isolated setting where drugs are used into the familiar setting of a bar, and from there into the professional and productive workplace, and finally into the privileged space of the home of an apparently well-to-do family. As the last man opens the door to his home and the camera shows his wife waiting for him, the voiceover warns that 'AIDS is closer than you think'. The audience is not the drug user, but the resident of the family home, and the rhetoric is not only moral but also spatial, reproducing the logic of the Pariolini who opposed the Casa famiglia in their neighbourhood park. The advert pays much more direct attention to the virus and to contagion than the Pariolini do, but both suggest – along with Donat-Cattin in his letter – that the upper-middle-class family and the space they inhabit stand farthest from a threat that looms ever nearer, and against which they must defend themselves. Donat-Cattin's letter of December 1988 and this advert from just over a year later show that those who campaigned against the Casa famiglia in late 1988 could draw upon messages created and disseminated by the state's central biomedical authority. A conflation of social and pathogenic contagion within biomedical discourse continued long beyond this period, though. *AIDS in Italia 20 anni dopo* was published in 2004 as a kind of updated version of *Il libro italiano dell'Aids*, published in 1994; both volumes were collaborations between the same three editors, Ferdinando Dianzani, Giuseppe Ippolito, and Mauro Moroni (discussed above), all well-known doctors who held a variety of positions in medical schools, government institutes, and non-governmental organisations in Italy and abroad. Chapter 7 of *AIDS in Italia 20 anni dopo* is entitled 'AIDS e tossicodipendenza' ('AIDS and drug addiction') and is written by Antonio Boschini and Camillo Smacchia. The introduction to the chapter closes thus: 'Even if in industrialised countries homosexuals represented the population most affected by HIV, drug users constituted a greater danger to public health, constituting a potential "bridge" for the spread of the epidemic to the general population via sexual means.'[31] Intravenous drug users are still depicted as a kind of conduit for the virus to pass from 'other' spaces and sections of society into the 'general population': the traditional family home and its members. Even within medical texts, those most at risk are characterised as a danger to others.[32]

'But Craxi's American declarations go too far': drug criminalisation

Fear of the sale and use of drugs was by no means limited to one upper-class neighbourhood of Rome.[33] The stigma associated with intravenous drug use was clearly stated in the title of an article in *La Repubblica* from 30 October 1988 – the same month that the Casa famiglia was originally slated to open. 'According to the majority of Italians, drug users should be punished', the headline declared. It went on to report that polls taken that month revealed that 57.6 per cent of Italians thought that both those who sold drugs as well as those who used them should face criminal charges; 24 per cent thought that the punishments should be the same for sellers and users. Eighty-four per cent said that they thought penalties for dealers were too lenient – 64 per cent said they thought a life sentence in prison was justified, while 8.5 per cent said they even supported the death penalty for those who sold drugs.[34]

These polls and their reporting in newspapers and in the first November issue of the popular Italian weekly *Panorama* magazine demonstrate a heightened social anxiety about drug use, but they did not emerge unprompted. October 1988 saw the visit of former Italian prime minister and leader of the Socialist Party Bettino Craxi to the USA. Before his arrival in Washington, DC, Craxi first travelled to New York and met with politicians including Rudolph Giuliani, then US Attorney for the Southern District of New York. Giuliani's efforts to 'clean up' New York City and push for tougher punishments for both drug dealers and users had influenced the work of Senator Alfonse D'Amato (Republican, New York) at the federal level. D'Amato was a vocal proponent of the Anti-Drug Abuse Act of 1988 (United States H.R.5210), a follow-up to the Anti-Drug Abuse Act of 1986. Introduced into the House of Representatives in August 1988 and passed there in September, the bill was reviewed, amended, and passed by the Senate in October, during the same weeks as Craxi's visit, before being presented to President Ronald Reagan, who signed it into law in early November. The bill centralised the federal government's efforts in the 'War on Drugs' with the creation of an Office of National Drug Control Policy within the Executive Office of the President. It also encouraged harsher punishments for drug traffickers, sellers, and users, including provisions for capital punishment for traffickers.[35]

As *La Repubblica* foreign correspondent Alberto Stabile explained in an article from 25 October 1988, it was exactly this climate of increased support for criminalisation and his exposure to the details of the American situation that inspired Craxi. According to Stabile, Craxi learnt most of all from his meeting with Giuliani.

At the end of this meeting, Craxi shared his own concerns about Italy. Stabile writes the following.

> The Italian situation, too, is an upsetting one; we risk finding ourselves in a country with South American characteristics. The secretary thus maintains that it is necessary to adjust the strategy and legislation against the trafficking of narcotics, not only making the penalties for traffickers more serious (up to a life sentence) but punishing users as well.[36]

Craxi would indeed begin a national conversation in Italy upon his return. 'Repressive measures to contain the spread of drugs in our country', said the anchor of the evening newscast on 3 November 1988, 'are those proposed by Bettino Craxi in the national meeting held symbolically in Palermo, capital of a region tormented by the mafia, the great entrepreneur in the trafficking of narcotics'.[37] The visual footage showed Craxi speaking at the Italian Socialist Party's annual meeting in Palermo, a meeting dedicated precisely to the topic of the War on Drugs and the new legislative measures Craxi had in mind to propose. As Craxi himself said, and as was transmitted during that broadcast, he sought:

> harsher penalties for big traffickers, up to a life sentence. I am talking about the organisers and disseminators of death who cannot but face the most severe penalty provided for by our changes. Harsher punishments for traffickers and dealers, an end to the regime founded upon the liberty to take drugs, and founded upon the possibility of taking advantage of the so-called small quantity. What is necessary are measures that have the capacity to dissuade, and the value of moral condemnation.

Craxi was blunt about the moral facet of his argument, and also that the Italian situation, as he saw it, should become part of broader international efforts to curb drug sale and use. 'All of Italy is at risk', the news anchor reported as Craxi's view, 'and the organised crime that lives off the market of death threatens to compromise the very foundations of democracy and of the economy, and of tarnishing, with its violence, the image and the position that the country is trying to retain in the international community'. Craxi made it plain that these measures were to do not only with crime and drug use, but also with Italy's image on the international stage. His claim that 'global measures are necessary' echoed American rhetoric, just as his proposed measures echoed the recent American legislative steps, and several journalists were quick to accuse Craxi of adopting a drastic American approach, of political posturing, and of appealing to more pernicious threads of public opinion in an effort to woo larger swaths of voters.[38]

Craxi's adoption of American rhetoric and American-influenced policies is in many ways unsurprising, particularly after his meetings with Giuliani. A television segment from 24 October 1988, when Craxi was still in New York, showed the two of them outside Giuliani's office, smiling for photographs and questions.[39] In a reference to Giuliani's Italian-American heritage, the news anchor spoke of the 'pizza connection' between the two countries and also their fight against organised crime families that specialised in drug trafficking. 'Greeting the honourable Craxi', continues the anchor, 'Giuliani said he had always had maximum collaboration from the Italian government, a collaboration that America points to as a model when it is requested from other nations. Craxi responded assuring the continuation of such cooperation, essential most of all in the War on Drugs.' Craxi's reference in Palermo ten days later to the image that Italy had to maintain on the world stage was likely a direct reference to Giuliani's characterisation of Italy as a model for cooperation with America in its War on Drugs.

This position did not go unchallenged. As US Attorney for the Southern District of New York, Giuliani had developed a reputation as a strict rule-enforcer with a particularly aggressive approach to drugs and to organised crime, and thus constituted an important alibi for Craxi's attempts to frame his proposals first and foremost as anti-mafia measures. However, some journalists immediately challenged Craxi's argument that these stricter measures, and particularly the criminalisation of drug consumption, constituted a way to fight the mafia. Some, like Gian Luigi Gessa, argued precisely the opposite: that not the criminalisation but rather the legalisation of heroin would deal the biggest blow to organised crime, since it would 'take away from the mafia the black market and related profits, and from the user the need to procure drugs through crime'.[40] 'Mafia families', added Miriam Mafai, 'and the big organised crime groups make unimaginable profits off this trafficking'.[41] Mafai agreed with Craxi that 'extremely severe punishments for drug traffickers' were worthwhile, but saw the criminalisation of drug use as an entirely separate issue: 'Craxi's taking up of a position in favour of punishments, for now unspecified, with regard to users as well, is surprising because it signals a total inversion of lay, socialist thought; of a culture, that is, that has had the merit of removing from the realm of blame and giving legitimacy to behaviours that before were considered deviant or even criminal.' Writing in the same newspaper the day before, Daniele Mastrogiacomo defended the existing law. 'Not punishing the user is a measure of great civility', he argued, 'that allows for the concentration of forces on trafficking. Proposing the death penalty for dealers or extremely harsh penalties for mere occasional users is only propaganda ... In the current situation, it is preposterous to go back to criminalising the user.'[42]

Despite these concerns, the existing law regarding drug sale and use was replaced less than two years later in 1990 with Law 162/90, more commonly known as the Craxi–Jervolino–Vassalli Law, for its co-sponsorship by Craxi and Rosa Russo Jervolino, then minister of social affairs. Politician and magistrate Tullio Grimaldi, writing just a few years after the law's passage, explained from a juridical perspective why its attempt to criminalise drug use was doomed to fail.

> Punishing the user like the dealer means fostering the intertwining of categories that should be contrasted, and the inevitable creation of a complicity between them. The user, pushed ever further into secrecy, is led to cover for his provider, both to defend himself from incrimination and so as not to lose a source of supply. Why, then, has this strategy been chosen?[43]

The answer, as many felt, was that Craxi had imported American ideologies and solutions. These masqueraded as government intervention to combat the mafia and to address what many perceived as a significant social threat. Just as American laws and law enforcement ultimately targeted the country's poor and its minoritised populations, so too did their Italian counterparts. This phenomenon of addressing social insecurity with punitive measures that criminalise remains, as Loïc Wacquant makes clear, one of the constitutive gestures of the neoliberal state. There is, in Wacquant's words, 'a close link between the ascendancy of neoliberalism ... and the deployment of the punitive and pro-active law enforcement policies targeting street delinquency and the categories trapped in the margins and cracks of the new economic and moral order'.[44] Italians who used heroin, who were largely younger and poorer and were in dire need of services and information in relation to HIV/AIDS, were criminalised as part of Craxi's contribution to the global War on Drugs and ostensible fight against organised crime.

These legislative measures had particularly pernicious consequences with regard to HIV/AIDS in Italy. The criminalisation of drug use almost certainly discouraged individuals from seeking help, both with their potential addiction and with regard to HIV prevention measures. Fernando Aiuti, on both *Viaggio intorno all'uomo* and *Sotto tiro*, argued explicitly and repeatedly for individualised prevention, that is, information and resources based on the specific needs and practices of each person. The context of the late 1980s, in which the criminalisation of drug use was very much on the cards, perhaps helps to explain Aiuti's relative silence on the issue of 'individualised prevention' for intravenous drug users. In 1993, just three years after its passage, Law 162/90 underwent significant revision and amendment. Still, the damage at the cultural, legislative, and penal levels had been done; by 1995, nearly 13 per cent of persons in Italian prisons were HIV-positive.[45]

Conclusion

Now several decades into the HIV/AIDS epidemic, activists around the world are still advocating and fighting for the decriminalisation of HIV and its transmission, sex work, and, importantly, substance use.[46] As a new pandemic in the form of Covid-19 reshapes our world once again, many of these same activists are cautioning against calls for increased policing in the name of global safety or public health.[47] The case of the Villa Glori casa famigilia per malati di Aids, and the broader cultural and legal climate in late 1980s Italy of which it was one symptom, demonstrate just how integral criminalisation has been to the HIV/AIDS epidemic and why so much work remains to be done. The combination of American anti-drug legislation and global policing with the prejudices of one well-to-do neighbourhood in Rome also demonstrates that HIV/AIDS must always be understood at global but also national and local levels.

Notes

1 The park is now also home to a collection of contemporary sculptures and art installations. Originally intended as a temporary exhibition dedicated to the Villa Glori Casa famiglia per malati di AIDS, *Varcare la soglia* opened in 1997; it was subsequently decided that the installations would be permanent, and two more works were added in 2000. The collection, which includes works by Fabio Mauri, Jannis Kounellis, and Paolo Canevari, among others, was organised and curated by art historian Daniela Fonti. For more, see the exhibition catalogue: Daniela Fonti (ed.), *Varcare la soglia: Dieci artisti contemporanei a Villa Glori. Villa Glori, 24 giugno–30 settembre 1997* (Rome: DeLuca, 1997).
2 Mario Armellini, *Sulla frontiera dell'Aids: La battaglia di don Luigi di Liegro e di Villa Glori contro la "peste" della paura* (Dogliani: Sensibili alle foglie, 1999), pp. 49–50.
3 Armellini, *Sulla frontiera dell'Aids*, p. 50. This and subsequent translations into English are by the author, unless otherwise noted.
4 In *Villa Glori: Viaggio nelle risposte possibili all'Aids* (dir. Luigi Faccinia, 1989).
5 Ferdinando Dianzani, Giuseppe Ippolito, and Mauro Moroni (eds), *AIDS in Italia, 20 anni dopo* (Milan: Masson, 2004), p. 39.
6 Dianzani et al., *AIDS in Italia*, pp. 39–40. The authors further hypothesised that the relatively younger age of heroin users in these areas meant that they were more at risk, as they might be more likely to share needles as part of communal rather than private drug use.
7 For a contemporary discussion of Italy's belated reaction to the HIV/AIDS epidemic, see David Moss, 'AIDS in Italy: emergency in slow motion', in *Action on AIDS: national policies in comparative perspective*, ed. by Barbara A. Misztal and David Moss (New York: Greenwood Press, 1990), pp. 135–66. Moss was writing his chapter in late 1988, just as the events discussed in this chapter were unfolding.
8 Carmela Giglio, 'I Parioli contro l'ospizio AIDS. Un'oasi per bambini diventerà infrequentabile', *Il Tempo*, 2 October 1988, quoted in Armellini, *Sulla frontiera dell'Aids*, p. 51.
9 Accessed at the Rai Teche, Rome, identifier: F43904.
10 The National Association for the Fight against AIDS: www.anlaidsonlus.it/chi-siamo/ (accessed 4 May 2020).
11 Accessed at the Rai Teche, Rome, identifier: FF6051. On this edition of *Viaggio intorno all'uomo*, Zavoli hosted a number of other guests from a diverse array of fields, including Russo Iervolino, then minister of social affairs, who will resurface later in this chapter.
12 Accessed at the Rai Teche, Rome, identifier: F14589. While Aiuti was the sole interviewee for this episode, Conti interviewed di Liegro on

the same programme two weeks earlier for the year's inaugural *Sotto tiro* (1 January 1989), effectively placing the two men into dialogue. Accessed at the Rai Teche, Rome, identifier: F14613.
13 Giglio, 'I Parioli contro l'ospizio AIDS', quoted in Armellini, *Sulla frontiera dell'Aids*, p. 51.
14 Dino Martirano, 'Rivolta anti Aids: "Non vogliamo il centro per malati ai Parioli"', *Corriere della Sera*, 4 October 1988, p. 35. This interest in seeing inside the Casa famiglia to determine the suitability of facilities recurs again and again.
15 Armellini, *Sulla frontiera dell'Aids*, p. 51.
16 Martirano, 'Rivolta anti Aids'.
17 *Ibid*.
18 A few days after this article was published, at the residents' meeting at the Grand Hotel Ritz Roma, the secretary from the city's second district also suggested that Caritas should 'find a deserted country house, maybe on the Cassia Road, where the earth can be tilled'. This road started on the other side of the Tiber from the Villa Glori and led out of the city towards Tuscany. Such suggestions of alternative venues at some distance were common. See Armellini, *Sulla frontiera dell'Aids*, p. 54.
19 *Ibid*., p. 53.
20 *Ibid*.
21 *Ibid*.
22 A segment entitled 'Roma: Interviste ad abitanti quartiere Parioli su casa alloggio, all'interno del parco di Villa Glori', *Almanacco + TG1*, Rai 1, 14 October 1988, accessed at the Rai Teche, Rome, identifier: T88336/101.
23 Armellini, *Sulla frontiera dell'Aids*, p. 52.
24 *Ibid*.
25 The letter is reprinted in its entirety in Vittorio Angoletto, *La società dell'Aids: La verità su politici, medici, volontari e multinazionali durante l'emergenza* (Milan: Baldini & Castoldi, 2000), pp. 134–6.
26 See also Chapters 2 and 7 in this volume on the positioning of marginalised populations as both 'at risk' themselves, but also a risk to others.
27 Agnoletto, *La società dell'Aids*, p. 137.
28 *Ibid*.
29 *Ibid*.
30 The advert is available on YouTube: www.youtube.com/watch?v=k33ta6HBotc (accessed 4 May 2020).
31 Antonio Boschini and Camillo Smacchia, 'AIDS e tossicodipendenza', in *AIDS in Italia 20 anni dopo*, ed. by Ferdinando Dianzani, Giuseppe Ippolito, and Mauro Moroni (Milan: Masson, 2004), p. 39.

32 There is a similarly deafening silence on this issue in the episode of *Viaggio intorno all'uomo* discussed above. The programme does predominantly aim at dealing with questions regarding young people and their sexualities and sex lives, so it makes sense that HIV/AIDS is addressed in this light. But there is an entire segment on HIV/AIDS that lasts nearly twenty minutes, including a long introductory voiceover that states repeatedly the need for clear information and productive conversation about the epidemic that needs to come from a variety of sources: medical authorities, schools, television, and others. There is one single mention of intravenous drug users, by Dr Aiuti, who also positions them as a kind of 'point-of-origin' population, endangering a risk-free general population: 'The most dramatic thing is that about 20 per cent of these persons with AIDS will be, unfortunately, heterosexuals, that is, persons who did not contract the virus through homosexual encounters, and who are not drug users. Thus in Italy there is a particular emergency because the virus is also spreading among the persons not belonging to so-called at-risk categories.' Similarly, despite a five-minute segment about homosexuality that features a teenage boy coming out to his mother via his filmed testimony, there is no explicit discussion of homosexuality with regard to HIV/AIDS, despite all the various specialists on the programme.
33 The quote in the heading to this section is taken from Miriam Mafai, 'Se Craxi scopre la guerra alla droga', *La Repubblica*, 27 October 1988.
34 'Per la maggioranza degli italiani, i tossicodipendenti vanno puniti', *La Repubblica*, 30 October 1988, p. 3.
35 It is available online: www.govtrack.us/congress/bills/100/hr5210/summary (accessed 8 May 2020).
36 Alberto Stabile, 'Puniamo i drogati', *La Repubblica*, 25 October 1988, p. 15.
37 *Almanacco + TG1*, Rai 1, accessed at the Rai Teche, Rome, identifier: T88308/101.
38 Miriam Mafai was perhaps clearest and most direct about this, in 'Se Craxi scopre la guerra alla droga', *La Repubblica*, 27 October 1988, p. 1.
39 *TG2 1945 + TG2 Lo Sport*, Rai 2, 24 October 1988, accessed at the Rai Teche, Rome, identifier: T88298/601.
40 Gian Luigi Gessa, 'L'eroina di stato', *La Repubblica*, 23 October 1988, p. 8.
41 Mafai, 'Se Craxi scopre la guerra alla droga', p. 9.
42 Daniele Mastrogiacomo, 'Ma i veri nemici sono i trafficanti', *La Repubblica*, 26 October 1988.
43 Tullio Grimaldi, 'La repressione penale aiuta il tossicodipendente', in *Il sistema droga. La costruzione sociale della tossicodipendenza*, ed. by Luisella De Cataldo Neuberger (Milan: Cedam, 1993), p. 311.

44 Loïc Wacquant, *Punishing the poor: the neoliberal government of social insecurity* (Durham, NC: Duke University Press, 2009), p. 1.
45 See UNAIDS, *Prisons and AIDS: UNAIDS point of view* (Geneva: UNAIDS, 1997); Claudio Mercandino, 'Carcere di Torino: Aids uccide ancora', *La Repubblica*, 25 February 1995, p. 20; and the *World prison brief* from the Institute for Crime & Justice Policy Research: https://prisonstudies.org/country/italy (accessed 8 May 2020). I thank Janet Weston for sharing these statistics and sources with me.
46 See, for example, Jason Rosenberg, 'Decriminalizing sex work, HIV, and substance use is the HIV prevention strategy we need', *The Body*, 8 April 2020: www.thebody.com/article/dasp-decriminalization-as-prevention (accessed 8 May 2020).
47 For example, see ACT UP NY on Twitter: https//twitter.com/actupny (accessed 8 May 2020).

3

Responding to HIV/AIDS in European prisons, 1980s–2000s

Janet Weston

The impact of HIV/AIDS on prisons (and vice versa) has received minimal attention within histories of the epidemic. Yet, researchers agree that 'HIV hit prisons early and it hit them hard'.[1] Prisons were flagged as locations of concern very early on. Their residents, like other already-marginalised groups whose lives became entangled with HIV/AIDS, became a source of anxiety among policy-makers and the media alike. Injecting drug use before and during incarceration, sex between men in prison, violence among inmates and towards staff, overcrowding and bad hygiene, and the poor general health of many of those behind bars were all highlighted as factors potentially contributing to the rapid spread of disease.[2] This, coupled with concern about the provision of adequate clinical and palliative care for prisoners affected by HIV/AIDS and possible infringements of their rights, prompted international organisations to gather information and issue specific recommendations for HIV/AIDS and prisons in 1987–8.[3] Such recommendations emphasised education, integration of people with HIV/AIDS into normal prison life, special efforts to avoid stigma and discrimination, and the need for services and standards of healthcare within prisons to match those existing elsewhere in the community.

Despite these clear recommendations, policy and practice in prisons remained the object of criticism throughout the 1990s and into the 2000s.[4] These ongoing concerns, along with some elements of secrecy and stigma adhering to prisons, help to explain why prisons and their occupants have featured little in histories of HIV/AIDS; successful activism, charismatic leadership, and a clear trajectory of change is difficult to locate. Researchers from contemporary and historical perspectives alike have ascribed the lack of agreement and action in the 1980s and 1990s regarding prisons and HIV/AIDS to the fact that medicine occupied an unusual position in this setting. As Virginia Berridge has argued with reference to the UK, fields in which the role of medicine was uncertain, including the insurance industry and drug addiction services as well as prisons, tended to struggle to agree and implement policies on HIV/AIDS.[5] Across Europe, prison medicine was isolated from mainstream medical services and public health, managed instead by departments of justice. Prison medicine was also closely involved in matters of discipline, approving individuals for punishments, special diets, or particular forms of work, and it traditionally adhered to local rather than national guidelines. In combination, these factors meant that the national and international policy consensus on HIV/AIDS, which was strongly influenced by medical and public health expertise, struggled to find purchase within prisons.

This chapter uses international evaluations and research from the 1980s, 1990s, and 2000s, along with media coverage, parliamentary debate, and oral histories, to develop these insights. It begins with a review of prison policy relating to HIV/AIDS across Western Europe, setting this against the guidelines and recommendations emerging from the World Health Organization (WHO) and Council of Europe. This reveals that many regions, if not most, did make efforts to meet international standards, especially from the 1990s onwards. Initial reactions to HIV/AIDS within prisons were often far from ideal, however, with widespread practices of segregation and breaches of medical confidentiality. In later years, particular sticking points were the provision of condoms and sterile injecting equipment to those in prison. A closer examination of two contrasting national responses, from the Republic of Ireland and Switzerland, helps to shed light on the reasons for national variation. International recommendations and activities were influential and could help those working towards change, but they could not override the broader national context within which prisons operated.

By highlighting the impact of HIV/AIDS on drug users and addiction services, this chapter forms part of recent attention to healthcare within prisons in the past, as well as gaps in our understanding of the history of HIV/AIDS.[6] The impact of HIV/AIDS on drug treatment has been widely recognised within the field

84   *Histories of HIV/AIDS in Western Europe*

of addiction research, but has slipped out of sight within mainstream HIV/AIDS histories.[7] Those who injected drugs, and who often faced unemployment, poverty, homelessness, incarceration, and poor health unrelated to HIV/AIDS, were dramatically affected by the epidemic. So, too, were their families, and the volunteers and professionals that provided services and care. Their omission from these mainstream histories threatens a second form of marginalisation. Activism also took a different form in the context of addiction work and prisons, and has not typically been included within the traditional roster of HIV/AIDS protest and direct action – with a few exceptions.[8] Action often demanded a very low profile, with staff discreetly bending or putting pressure on official rules to generate practical or policy change. More public action was led by individuals at some personal risk but, as with hidden prison activism, its impact was rarely obvious or clear-cut. The example of prisons suggests that HIV/AIDS activism should be conceived more broadly, to incorporate covert action, activities that tested professional boundaries, and individual risk-taking, even when those actions did not prompt immediate or obvious change. Interventions to improve policies or conditions concerning HIV/AIDS and prisons rarely made the headlines and were not always successful, as the case studies of Switzerland and the Republic of Ireland show. First, though, we should consider the international recommendations for prisons that emerged in the late 1980s, and the extent to which these were adopted and resisted.

International recommendations and their implementation

The WHO Special Programme on AIDS held its first consultation on HIV/AIDS in prisons in November 1987, as did the Council of Europe's Social and Health Affairs Committee. Both bodies issued their initial recommendations soon thereafter. These were very similar to each other, emphasising the need for education for staff and prisoners about HIV/AIDS, voluntary rather than mandatory testing, and full integration of prisoners with HIV/AIDS into standard prison routines rather than any form of segregation. They also recommended the provision of condoms to prisoners, and, in more cautious terms, careful consideration of whether to provide sterile injecting equipment to prisoners in some circumstances.[9] The transmission of HIV within prisons via injecting drug use was addressed more forcefully in 1993, when further consultations on the situation in prisons prompted more comprehensive guidelines.[10] These were emphatic in recommending an absolute ban on compulsory HIV testing of prisoners, and highlighted prisoners' rights to healthcare, 'including preventive measures, equivalent to that available in the community'. Drawing special attention to the realities of HIV transmission within prisons, 'notably needle sharing among injecting drug users and unprotected sexual intercourse', the 1993 recommendations reiterated the need for condoms to be made available and called more definitively for the provision of disinfectant and clean injecting equipment inside prisons in countries where these were available to non-incarcerated drug users.

These recommendations reflected the broader international policy consensus that eventually emerged in response to HIV/AIDS, which favoured education, voluntarism, and the minimisation of harms and was sensitive (at least in theory) to the implications of discrimination and inequality. International recommendations were significant not only for setting standards and expectations, but also because their production generated some of the only pan-European data on HIV/AIDS in prisons. Figures gathered by the Council of Europe in 1987–8 showed that only Spain had so far identified significant numbers of people in prison with HIV/AIDS, but there was a clear belief that other countries would quickly follow suit.[11] By the mid-1990s, Italy, Spain, Scotland, and Berlin had the highest known rates of HIV infection within their incarcerated populations, with data from Denmark, France, and the Netherlands also indicating that a significant proportion of their prison populations may be affected.[12] Italy, it was reported, faced the highest numbers in Europe; in 1995, its prisons housed some 7,500 individuals with HIV/AIDS.[13] Extremely low figures, which may have reflected low rates of HIV testing as much as prevalence, were reported from most of Southeastern Europe. Of particular concern for Western Europe was the fact that rates of HIV infection appeared to be so much higher within prisons than in the general population; small studies from France and Switzerland suggested rates between 50 and 200 per cent higher, and researchers regularly pointed out that most people were in prison for a short time only and therefore presented a risk to the wider public upon their release.[14] Many prison administrations in Western Europe had been spurred into action in 1985, when a test for HIV became available. Confirmed cases of HIV prompted an element of panic at this time, within prisons as elsewhere in society. Overcrowding and unhygienic conditions within most prisons, combined with concerns among staff about anything that might disrupt good order and control, meant that anxiety within prisons about HIV/AIDS was particularly intense. In some locations, including the Republic of Ireland and Scotland, prisoners diagnosed as or even simply suspected of being HIV-positive were immediately released.[15] In England, all movement in or out of one prison was temporarily halted in an attempt to create a localised quarantine.[16] In Norway, the situation in Oslo's prison was briefly 'turbulent', with some prisoners successfully demanding the separation and isolation of those among them testing positive for HIV.[17] In Belgium, pressure came from staff; a threatened strike in December 1985 led to the creation of an 'AIDS ward' in one prison, where the five prisoners known to have HIV were to be housed.[18] This practice of segregation in a separate wing or unit was also adopted in the Republic of Ireland and Portugal, and later in Greece, Sweden, and Bulgaria as well.[19] In 1987, only six countries reported no special restrictions at all on the accommodation, movement, or activities of prisoners with HIV/AIDS: Austria, Denmark, France, Italy, Spain, and Switzerland.[20]

It is notable that these decisions to implement special restrictions or separate units were often driven by direct action in various forms. Those in prison – inmates and staff alike – expressed their demands in relation to HIV/AIDS, and the resultant or threatened disorder was sometimes sufficient for those demands to be met. Given that these demands tended to favour discrimination and segregation, they might find little sympathy today, but they are nonetheless part of the picture of direct action inspired by HIV/AIDS. It is also notable that locations avoiding special restrictions included those with the highest rates of HIV/AIDS among their prison populations. This suggests that known prevalence had a significant impact on responses to HIV/AIDS within prisons. Paradoxically, perhaps, a small number of confirmed cases of HIV/AIDS was more likely to provoke extreme reactions than large numbers of diagnoses. Segregating a handful of individuals was easy, and in fact a natural solution to the perceived problem. Most prison systems already featured separate institutions, wings, units, or cells for particular types of inmate. Individuals could also be isolated for their own safety or the safety of others, or in the interests of discipline. Resources and procedures were therefore already in place for separating out a new classification of prisoner – those with HIV/AIDS. But segregating or putting special measures into place for much larger numbers, or large proportions of the total prison population, was much more difficult in practical terms.

First reactions tended to have a long afterlife. In many of the countries where segregation for prisoners with HIV/AIDS was initially adopted, this practice outlasted initial waves of panic by some margin. Segregation could quickly become a new norm, justified in the interests of good order as well as safety. The existence of a separate 'HIV unit' was challenged but upheld by the Belgian courts in 1989, although the unit was closed the following year after ministerial intervention. A separate unit survived in Dublin well into the 1990s, as discussed below.[21] Even where there was no formal policy of segregating all prisoners with HIV/AIDS, it was not unusual for segregation to be permitted more widely than official guidelines implied. Policy in England and Wales as well as in Norway followed this line, allowing segregation of individuals with HIV/AIDS on a case-by-case basis. This permissive policy engendered rather different outcomes in the two locations, with some English prisons developing their own informal policies of blanket segregation, while evidence from Norway suggests that segregation was used rarely, if at all.[22]

Segregation was criticised for creating a false sense of security, and for acting as a powerful disincentive to HIV testing. Officially, policies on HIV testing quickly fell into line with the overwhelming international consensus that testing must be voluntary, but in the prison context the line between voluntary and compulsory was often blurred. Anyone refusing an HIV test in a Luxembourgian prison, for example, was placed in isolation, and the same applied in some English prisons. Wandsworth Prison in London maintained a separate 'Viral Infection Restriction Unit' for prisoners considered to be 'high-risk' who had refused an HIV test, as well as those already diagnosed, until at least 1995.[23] In Germany, mandatory tests were still permitted in Bavaria as late as 1994, and elsewhere 'those who refuse are treated as if they were HIV positive until tested', meaning that in practice very few did refuse.[24] Cyprus, Italy, and Spain all reported the impressive fact that not one single prisoner from an 'at-risk group' had refused to undergo a test, which raises some questions about how voluntary these tests really were.[25] This is also indicative of persistent stigmatisation and discrimination within prisons on the basis of known or suspected HIV status, not fully captured in official policy and reports.[26]

By the early 1990s, the importance of educating staff and prisoners to reduce risky behaviour and stigma alike was widely accepted, and almost all European prison systems were providing information about HIV/AIDS via multiple media. The only known exceptions were two German states, both formerly in the German Democratic Republic (GDR), where no cases of HIV or AIDS had been identified among prisoners and the need for information on the subject was still denied.[27] Elsewhere, though, innovative methods of providing information to prisoners were reported, including theatrical productions, posters designed by fellow inmates, and quizzes with prizes. Dedicated HIV/AIDS teams had been established in many locations; a special team of medical and disciplinary staff was set up at Saughton Prison in Scotland, for example, to provide education and counselling.[28] Such efforts were not without problems of their own. One issue, mentioned only rarely in the 1990s, was that a small but significant number of prisoners across Europe did not speak the local language to a high standard and would not benefit from standardised education programmes. Others, it was suggested, might need interventions tailored to particular cultural backgrounds and beliefs, as well as languages. In 1993 in Amsterdam, an external welfare organisation delivered information to groups of Turkish and Moroccan prisoners in their first language and without prison staff present, which reportedly allowed for more open discussion and better results than the usual education sessions, but this remained a rarity.[29] Similarly, information and services tailored to the needs of women and young people in prison were flagged in the 1990s as having received very little attention, but remained slow to develop.[30] Despite these criticisms, education was one area, at least, where widespread efforts were in evidence and good intentions (if not always good delivery) were generally praised.

Much more controversial was the issue of condoms for those in prison. In 1986, condoms were reportedly available in a small number of prisons, in parts of Switzerland and possibly also Spain, but a swift rejection of the idea in both France and Britain was a cause for concern.[31] However, within a few years French policy had reversed, and 'initial refusal on legal grounds has been replaced by a policy of availability on public health grounds' in 1988.[32] Other nations gradually followed suit, sometimes propelled by prisoners' demands. In Germany, for example, a prisoner strike in 1992 led to scrutiny of the status quo concerning HIV/AIDS, followed by a pilot study for providing condoms.[33] By the mid-1990s a significant minority of countries were still insistent on their refusal to provide condoms to prisoners under any circumstances, including in open prisons (where inmates have limited supervision and can leave the prison for work or education) or on release, including Bulgaria, Cyprus, former GDR states, Iceland, Ireland, and across the UK.[34] Even where official policy had become permissive, practice was variable. In the Netherlands, condoms were officially available, but this was overshadowed by emphatic prohibitions on sex between men in prison and few prisoners ever asked for them. At one Dutch prison, they were not available at all because the governor objected.[35] A similar pattern of variability, often depending on individual governors or doctors, was reproduced in England and Wales when policy changed to become more permissive in the mid-1990s.[36]

The prisoners' strike in Germany is a rare example of direct action on the part of prisoners that saw positive results. More commonly, such activism in support of the wider distribution of condoms was not wholly successful and is now little-known. Glen Fielding's efforts are typical in this respect. Fielding had been imprisoned in England, and after being refused condoms he used the courts (and associated publicity) to try to generate a change in policy – a protracted form of action that outlasted his prison sentence but did not end in definitive success. The court held that the policy of the prison service had been misinterpreted in Fielding's case, but that it was itself lawful. This was reported in some quarters as a victory, but for those involved it was a partial disappointment, and its impact on the prison service, if any, was unclear.[37]

More controversial even than condoms was the question of services for those injecting drugs while in prison. This mirrored hesitation in the wider community, where 'harm-reduction' approaches, such as the prescribing of opioid substitutes like methadone or the provision of clean injecting equipment or disinfectant and advice on safer injecting, were introduced in a much slower and more piecemeal fashion than condoms and messages about safer sex. Denmark had begun to provide sterile needles to prisoners by 1992, but only on release and only if used equipment had been confiscated upon detention.[38] The Swiss prison system was the first in Europe to offer a needle exchange programme within its prison establishments, as will be discussed in more detail below. Early experimentation began in several Swiss prisons in around 1992 and was formalised a few years later. Success there was persuasive in the mid-1990s for some prisons in Germany, as well as elsewhere in Switzerland.[39] But these remained the exception rather than the rule; as of 2018, within Western Europe only Switzerland, Germany, Luxembourg, and Spain offered any needle exchange programmes at all for those in prison.[40]

The provision of disinfectants to allow prisoners to clean their injecting equipment was slightly more popular. 'Hygiene kits' including disinfectant and instructions on cleaning syringes had been introduced into some Swiss and Catalan prisons as early as the late 1980s.[41] By 1992, disinfectant was also available in Belgium, Luxembourg, the Netherlands, Spain, and some prisons in Denmark, France, and Germany as well. Scotland was then spurred into action by confirmation that HIV transmission had occurred within one of its prisons, Glenochil, in 1993, and began to provide sterilising tablets alongside information about the risks of injecting.[42] Localised and informal efforts to provide disinfectant were also attempted in the Republic of Ireland, as discussed below, but here, as in England and Wales, such efforts struggled to take root. A pilot scheme for disinfecting tablets was run in England in the late 1990s and received a positive evaluation, but a wider roll-out was delayed and then implemented in only a few locations.[43]

Overall, then, it took time for international recommendations to be translated into practice within prison settings, and some recommendations remained unmet. In the mid-1990s, two leading researchers concluded pessimistically that 'clear guidelines from international organisations carry little weight in the context of the security dominated world of penal systems', and were 'largely ignored'.⁴⁴ This overview, borne of frustration at the slow progress being made with harm-reduction initiatives within prisons, overlooked many of the positive effects that international recommendations had already had – particularly concerning education, integration, and, to a lesser but still significant extent, the provision of condoms. Prisons also continued to move towards ever greater adherence to these guidelines as the 1990s progressed.

Numerous barriers to faster and more fulsome compliance were identified, including a lack of awareness or resources, the weakness of prison medicine, especially within an environment that prioritised security and control over health, and national laws or local rules that stood in the way. The controversial nature of some of the recommendations was also acknowledged as a factor.⁴⁵ These issues all played their part, but as the case studies of Switzerland and the Republic of Ireland show, what was perhaps even more influential in determining how prison systems responded to HIV/AIDS was the broader context of prison management, addiction work, and public health within which prison policies on HIV/AIDS had to operate. The profile of the HIV/AIDS epidemic and the prison populations in these two countries was similar, with injecting drug use featuring prominently. Both also had relatively small prison populations, and of course they were presented with the same international and European guidelines. But while Switzerland became a trailblazer in harm-minimisation approaches in the late 1980s and 1990s, setting the scene for equally radical efforts within its prisons, changes in the Republic of Ireland are harder to detect. International guidance and the exchange of ideas across borders could inspire at the individual level but required the right local context before they could truly take root.

Irish and Swiss prisons: a comparison

When HIV/AIDS emerged in the Republic of Ireland, it was largely viewed as part of the growing problem of injecting drug use. Addiction to heroin had been attracting some attention and concern within medical circles since the early 1980s, following a very rapid increase in the numbers of young people in Dublin identified as heroin users and experiencing serious health problems.[46] A national committee was set up to address this in early 1985, and by the time of its first report a year later, HIV/AIDS was one of its key areas of interest.[47] References to HIV/AIDS and prisons were first uttered in the Dáil Éireann (parliamentary assembly) as part of this wider discussion about heroin addiction, and inmates with HIV/AIDS were universally characterised as drug users by officials and family members alike.[48] Homosexuality remained illegal in the Republic of Ireland until 1993, and this along with the influence of the Church over matters of sexuality and health may have made it easier for individuals and policy-makers to attribute HIV/AIDS to drug use rather than sex, potentially distorting the epidemiological picture. As one addiction worker later remarked, 'everybody found it much easier to talk about drug use and injecting than safer sex'.[49] Nevertheless, research from the early 1990s showed that a 'substantial proportion of Ireland's total HIV-infected population have spent time in custody in Mountjoy prison' in Dublin, placing this prison and its actions at the heart of Ireland's HIV/AIDs epidemic.[50]

The issue of HIV/AIDS in Irish prisons erupted in late 1985. The first diagnosis of HIV within a prison was made in October, after a prisoner requested a test, and was handled poorly.[51] By January 1986 around fifty individuals in Mountjoy's male and female prisons – comfortably over 10 per cent of the prison's population – had been identified as HIV-positive.[52] An 'official party' urgently visited Britain to 'see at first hand what steps were being taken to deal with prisoners found to be HTLV III positive' there. Irish prison staff also reportedly received information about this new health crisis from prison medical officers to allay their concerns.[53] However, at this time there were no full-time prison medical officers in the country and no nursing staff at all; 'prison medical officers' were a handful of GPs who would visit prisons on a part-time basis and were held in very low regard.[54] This calls into question the quality of any information received by prison staff, and makes their reaction to HIV/AIDS less surprising. Staff, through the Prison Officers' Association, placed pressure on prison administrators to segregate those with HIV/AIDS. Doctors shared the identities of those testing positive with prison management, and after an unsuccessful attempt to house this group in an alternative prison on the outskirts of the city, an area of Mountjoy already used for segregation was adopted for those with HIV/AIDS in 1986.

By 1987, 136 prisoners in the Republic of Ireland had been identified as HIV-positive.[55] Segregation continued, despite concerns over suicides and reports of poor mental health among those held in segregation, particularly as deaths from AIDS-related conditions began to occur. But among staff and prisoners alike, many remained unwilling to countenance reintegration. Segregation had encouraged a belief in all quarters that those with HIV/AIDS presented serious risks to the general prison population. For those held in the separate unit, their special status meant that they could receive extra foods and welfare services, including access to a different doctor who had a particular interest in HIV/AIDS, all of which might be lost if they returned to normal accommodation.[56] Any attempt to reintegrate prisoners with HIV/AIDS would therefore be met with protest from all quarters. The Irish prison service was not blind to this problem and the inflexibility of its staff, and submitted a request to the Council of Europe for 'information from Member States on the problems caused by AIDS in prisons and the reactions of prison staff to the crisis'. This led to the Council's initial research and recommendations on the subject,[57] but change was slow to occur in the Irish prison system. Although more vocal criticisms of the prison service's response in general, and the segregation unit in particular, began to emerge, the segregation unit was not fully disbanded until 1995 – making it one of the last of its kind in Western Europe.[58]

Alongside the problem of segregation and the associated lack of medical confidentiality for those with HIV/AIDS in prison, the issue of drug addiction continued and grew. In the community, services began to favour methods of harm-minimisation, including the provision of sterile needles and longer-term prescribing of methadone, but this was somewhat tentative and covert[59] and had little direct impact within prisons until the late 1990s.[60] Yet, as community services began to change, doctors and addiction workers did not ignore the needs of drug users in prison – not least because prison was a semi-regular aspect of many of their service users' lives.[61] When steps were taken to bring the European Peer Support

Project (EPSP) to Dublin, its organisers were keen to include prison officers and former prisoners for this reason. The EPSP exemplifies the international networks and conversations that sprang up around addiction in response to HIV/AIDS, but events in Ireland demonstrate their limited impact on prisons where local conditions were not right.

The EPSP began in 1993, inspired by self-organisation among drug users in the Netherlands.[62] This had suggested the potential for peer support to improve the health and wellbeing of drug users. The EPSP was funded by the European Commission and aimed to 'encourage, develop, and support professional drug aid services and drug-user self-organizations and networks to start or extend peer support strategies, especially in the field of AIDS prevention'.[63] As part of the second phase of this programme, which focused on European regions where peer support was not yet developed, a three-day seminar was held for prison staff, statutory addiction workers, voluntary workers, and drug users in Dublin in late 1995.[64] This was jointly coordinated and led by Dutch and Irish addiction specialists, who sought out a range of participants, including those from the prison staff who were 'sitting on the fence': not already persuaded of the value of peer support or harm-reduction approaches, and not adamant that they were doomed to fail. Many of the drug user participants and prison staff knew each other from the prison setting, leading to some tension and hostility at the outset, but over the three days 'there was a lot of learning' and, 'by the end of it, that business of "You're a human being too"' began to emerge.[65]

The seminars addressed attitudes, myths, and realities around drug use, and the risks of HIV and hepatitis, combining education with personal storytelling to encourage awareness of different perspectives and experiences. Dutch participants also shared their experience of initiatives such as needle exchanges, generating discussion and, in one participant's view, a new 'openness' among Irish prison staff to these ideas. Prison staff reported feeling safer in their work as a result of the seminars, having come to appreciate where the risks lay, the kinds of experiences that drug users encountered, and what could be done to help reduce dangers to everyone. After the seminar, thanks to the interest and enthusiasm of one or two officers in particular, participants (including drug users) were invited to deliver training on safer injecting and blood-borne viruses to prison staff on four or five occasions.

To illustrate the kind of changes in approach and attitude that this initiative brought about, one participant recalled the feedback she had received. 'One prison officer said to me ... before he did the training, if he approached a cell and saw someone starting to inject, he would've gone in to interrupt and to stop that injecting. He was asked the question [during the training] why, because you're not going to stop their drug use, and he'd never thought of it like that.' Afterwards, he reflected that 'I would now be saying to my colleagues close the door, and let them finish, because we're more at risk if we make them stop because that person is so desperate' (Ibid.). Recognition of the realities and risks of injecting drug use brought about these modest examples of attitudinal and practical change. Community workers began to hear that those in prison had more confidence in certain officers – particularly those who had undertaken the training – and would feel able to turn to them with any concerns. Notably, some staff began covertly leaving quantities of disinfectant or extra spoons around their prison, and taking time to check the wellbeing of particular individuals known to be injecting.[66] These could be included as forms of HIV/AIDS activism, albeit ones that were necessarily covert or at least discreet, given the particular context of the prison environment.

The long-term consequences of the EPSP in Ireland were significant. The Union for Improved Services, Communication and Education was set up to represent the interests of drug users in Ireland, emulating similar organisations elsewhere, and for many of the individual participants it was a transformative experience. Yet, initiatives such as providing disinfectant within prisons relied on the presence and energy of a small number of people who soon moved on in their careers. Some elements of this harm-minimisation approach may have survived within prison cultures, encouraged by broader shifts in services and standards, but official policy on disinfectant and needle exchanges remained unmoved. The idea of enabling safer injecting within Irish prisons is still sufficiently controversial for some of those involved in the mid-1990s to want to remain anonymous. This was not a form of activism or international exchange with a clear or rapid trajectory of success.

One former prison doctor in Dublin, reflecting on the 1990s, recalled seeing 'a lot of discussion in the media in the world about needle exchanges, in Geneva or Zurich, but it was never relevant to Ireland'.[67] Switzerland became a high-profile pioneer in harm-reduction initiatives in the 1990s, and its story was indeed markedly different from the Irish example. HIV/AIDS hit Switzerland particularly hard and, as in the Republic of Ireland, its epidemic was closely associated with injecting drug use. By 1992, Switzerland (along with Italy) was said to have 'the highest cumulative incidence of AIDS cases in Europe, long established drug markets, and a substantial percentage of AIDS cases accounted for by drug use'.[68] The first reports of prisoners with HIV emerged in late 1985 from Basel-Stadt, and soon it seemed that something like 10 per cent of those in prison were affected.[69] In contrast with the Irish case, though, practices of segregation did not follow these diagnoses. This is not to say that fear and attempts at quarantine were entirely absent; there is some evidence of hostile reactions to individuals thought to be infected, and steps to separate them from the general prison population or to ban, for example, those with HIV/AIDS from work in prison kitchens.[70] Yet, these initial sparks of panic do not seem to have solidified into general policy or practice.

The number or proportion of prisoners affected by HIV/AIDS does not seem to explain this variation, as both locations saw similar prevalence rates. Three differences between the prison systems of these countries stand out as potentially relevant. First, segregation had been practised fairly commonly in Mountjoy Prison in the 1970s in dealing with political prisoners, meaning that the facilities and a culture to support segregation were already in place there. Second, the first volunteers for HIV tests from Swiss prisons included staff as well as inmates, suggesting that information about HIV transmission and testing was provided to both groups in a more formal capacity and on an equal footing. This might also mean that there were plans in place in the event of positive test results, whereas in Dublin the impetus for testing came from inmates themselves and the prison administration was entirely unprepared.

Last, it also appears that Swiss prison medical personnel were less willing to serve the demands of prison management than their Irish counterparts. In late 1985, a doctor at Thorberg prison in the canton of Bern refused to report cases of AIDS to the management of their institution, citing the need to respect medical confidentiality, and subsequently resigned over the issue.[71] This public act – arguably a form of activism in itself – placed a spotlight on tensions between medical standards and prison demands, prompting questions in the Nationalrat (federal assembly) as to whether prison doctors could or should breach confidentiality in the specific context of HIV/AIDS in prisons. Subsequently, prison governors in Switzerland were at pains to stress that prison doctors would *not* share test results, suggesting that medical standards had won out on this occasion.[72] This may simply have been a question of personality, with one particularly vocal and independently minded doctor in Bern forcing the issue, and in so doing pushing policy-makers to give clear guidance. It may also indicate a medical service that was, as a whole, better informed about HIV/AIDS or more philosophically attuned to public health priorities over those of penal discipline. In either case, greater medical influence within Swiss prisons may well have steered managers away from any impulse to segregate.

In terms of drug addiction, Switzerland was an early adopter of harm-reduction approaches in the community. By the early 1990s it was at the cutting edge of harm-reduction initiatives, which were widely discussed and debated internationally. A needle exchange programme was launched in Zurich in 1988, where the majority of Swiss injecting drug use was to be found. This programme also supplied 'hygienic cotton swabs and vein creams, condoms, tea and fruit; it provided primary medical care, hepatitis-B vaccination and information on treatment options, as well as instruction in safe sex, hygiene and health behaviour'.[73] Methadone-prescribing programmes tripled between 1986 and 1990, and the prescribing of heroin was also trialled, although hindered by international controls on the importation of the drug. Out-patient services began to include 'street rooms' where injecting drug use under hygienic conditions, with showers and medical supervision, was tolerated.[74] Elements of these radical programmes were extended to Swiss prisons, including the 'hygiene kits' already mentioned, trials of heroin prescription, and methadone maintenance programmes in Basel, Bern, Geneva, and Zurich in the early 1990s.[75]

Swiss prisons also began to adopt syringe exchange programmes. In around 1992, at Oberschöngrün prison in Solothurn, a part-time medical officer who saw that many patients were clearly injecting drugs on a regular basis began to dispense sterile injecting equipment. When this was discovered, the governor of the prison reportedly 'listened to his arguments about prevention of transmission of HIV and hepatitis, as well as injection-site abscesses, and sought approval from the Cantonal authorities to sanction the distribution of sterile needles and syringes'. This was characterised by its supporters as a brave 'act of medical disobedience' on the part of the medical officer,[76] setting the stage for prisons elsewhere in the country to follow this lead. Where researchers and advocates saw admirable disobedience, historians might also see another atypical form of activism, enacted by both medical and disciplinary staff (just about) within professional boundaries but no less significant for that.

At around the same time, the medical staff at Hindelbank, a prison for women in the canton of Bern, began calling for a needle exchange programme. Staff reported high rates of needle sharing, and voluntary organisations may already have started to distribute syringes as an emergency response within the prison.[77] A formal pilot was launched in 1994, after several years spent winning support at the federal level in order to overcome cantonal opposition. The Federal Office of Health backed the scheme on the grounds that its own health strategy promised that those in prison would receive the same healthcare as those outside. The Federal Office of Justice was also involved, seeking and obtaining legal confirmation that a pilot could proceed.[78] The pilot included lectures, group lessons, counselling, and machines to dispense condoms and sterile injecting equipment. It was evaluated positively, and subsequently rolled out in Swiss and also German prisons.[79] By 1999, further pilots of vending machines to distribute sterile injecting equipment were still being rolled out across Swiss prisons, suggesting that acceptance and implementation was relatively slow, but still forthcoming.[80]

All this is not to say that the responses to HIV/AIDS within Swiss prisons at the end of the twentieth century were flawless, by any means. There was considerable regional variation, and even variation from prison to prison, with a minority of establishments adopting fulsome harm-reduction measures. (The criminalisation of HIV transmission in Switzerland raises its own concerns.) Nevertheless, Switzerland was frequently held up as a trailblazer in the field of HIV/AIDS prevention in prisons, and clearly followed a different path to the Irish prison service over the 1980s and

1990s. This was largely a reflection of the approach to addiction in wider community services, but that is not quite the whole story. Researchers in the 1990s argued that individual disobedience and a willingness to engage in 'courageous experiment' in Switzerland were the factors that changed prison policy, but Irish prison officers engaged in such disobedience and experimentation, particularly following their interactions with the EPSP, and this did not lead to nationally recognised pilot studies or changes in policy. Something was clearly different in Switzerland.

What stands out from these two case studies is the decentralisation (or otherwise) of prison management and the role of prison medical staff. The prison service was tightly centralised in Ireland, with all decisions flowing directly from the Department of Justice.[81] Policy change had to come from the top. In Switzerland, each of the twenty-six cantons managed its own prisons and made its own arrangements for healthcare, encouraging much greater independence. Regional variation could be more marked (and, as Hindelbank showed, regional government did not always support change), but local innovation was more likely. Innovation among medical personnel was particularly important, as medical expertise could be extremely influential. Disobedience among prison officers in Dublin could not change policy on the provision of disinfectant, but disobedience among doctors might have been different.[82] There is no reason to think that Irish prison doctors would have been less influential then their Swiss counterparts, and, indeed, one well positioned observer in Ireland felt strongly that the doctors she worked with in prisons could have demanded change.[83] The realisation of this influence was hindered by that tightly centralised system, as well as the broader picture of harm minimisation in the community.

Conclusion

By the late 1980s, both Switzerland and the Republic of Ireland faced a significant number of prisoners with HIV/AIDS, as did many other regions of Europe. The extent of HIV/AIDS within prisons was closely associated with the extent of injecting drug use, and the use of custodial sentences for drug-related offences. The adoption of international recommendations within prisons, particularly those concerning controversial harm-reduction measures such as needle exchanges, echoed harm-reduction initiatives in the wider community. Where harm-reduction measures had been adopted early and energetically in community healthcare, prisons were more likely to meet international guidelines regarding safer injecting, as in the case of Switzerland. In contrast, where harm reduction struggled to attain a foothold in community services, it remained unthinkable for prisons.

This does not mean that international recommendations focusing on prisons served no purpose. Pressure from international bodies such as the Council of Europe, and from critical reports drawing on these international standards, encouraged prisons away from practices of segregation and towards education and respect for confidentiality. Among those working in prisons, contact with European networks provided information and ideas, and sometimes prompted radical experimentation. This experimentation can be seen as a form of HIV/AIDS activism, albeit one that was not always successful. As the Irish and Swiss examples show, these experiments required medical endorsement and a responsive prison administration in order to flourish; the ways in which prison management was organised, just as much as prison healthcare, could have a significant impact.

This raises questions about what is included and remembered as HIV/AIDS activism. In the context of prisons, activism was often discreet and rarely met with immediate results. Sometimes, as with the prison doctor in Bern who resigned over confidentiality concerns, the result was not one single event or decision, and its impact is only detectable with hindsight. Perhaps inevitably, such actions have rarely been celebrated as examples of activism. The actions of Swiss prison doctors and public health workers in providing sterile injecting equipment are almost an exception, but these actions were carried out more or less within the boundaries of professional and expert decision-making. Can such actions be activism? A fuller history of HIV/AIDS may require our definitions of activism to expand to include those who tested such boundaries, who took decisions that were personally risky, who pressed their colleagues to do the same – and those who tried to do these things but failed. Nor was all activism within prison settings something to celebrate. Actions by prisoners and staff alike to demand the segregation of those with HIV could have negative and long-lasting consequences, but it was activism nonetheless.

Finally, these examples also begin to hint at some of the experiences of HIV/AIDS that have so far been largely overlooked and require much greater attention. For those working in the field of addiction or with communities affected by heroin use in the 1980s, HIV/AIDS brought enormous change. For injecting drug users and their families and friends, its toll was enormous and devastating. And for prisons across Europe, a new role in public health was formulated, resisted, and cautiously embraced.

Acknowledgements

The research for this chapter was funded by the Wellcome Trust as part of grant number 103341, 'Prisoners, Medical Care, and Entitlement to health in England and Ireland 1850–2000'. I am very grateful to Catherine Cox and Hilary Marland, the primary investigators on that project, for their encouragement and support and to colleagues at LSHTM's Centre for History in Public Health for their valuable comments on an earlier draft.

Notes

1 Ralf Jürgens, Manfred Nowak, and Marcus Day, 'HIV and incarceration: prisons and detention', *Journal of the International AIDS Society*, 14.26 (2011), p. 2.
2 Gary P. Wormser, 'Acquired immunodeficiency syndrome in male prisoners: new insights into an emerging syndrome', *Annals of Internal Medicine*, 98.3 (1983), 297; Theodore M. Hammett and Monique Sullivan, *AIDS in correctional facilities: issues and options* (Washington, DC: US Department of Justice, 1986); Timothy Harding and Georgette Schaller, 'HIV/AIDS policy for prisons or for prisoners?', in *AIDS in the World*, ed. by Jonathan M. Mann, Daniel J. M. Tarantola, and Thomas W. Netter (Cambridge, MA: Harvard University Press, 1992), pp. 761–9.
3 World Health Organization, *Statement from the consultation on prevention and control of AIDS in prisons* (Document number WHO/SPA/INF/87.14, Geneva, 16 November 1987); *Draft report*

on a coordinated European health policy to prevent the spread of AIDS in prison. Rapporteur: Mr Martino (Strasbourg: Council of Europe, 16 April 1988), available online at: https://rm.coe. int/16807ab00bpacecom074887.pdf (accessed 15 October 2019); Council of Europe, Parliamentary Assembly, *Recommendation 1080 on a coordinated European policy to prevent the spread of AIDS in prisons*, 30 June 1988, available from the University of Minnesota Human Rights Library online: www1.umn.edu/humanrts/instree/ recommendation1080.html (accessed 8 April 2016).

4 Timothy Harding, 'HIV infection and AIDS in the prison environment: a test case for the respect of human rights', in *AIDS and drug misuse: the challenge for policy and practice in the 1990s*, ed. by John Strang and Gerry V. Stimson (London; New York: Routledge, 1990), pp. 197–210; Harding and Schaller, 'HIV/AIDS policy for prisons or for prisoners?'; Heino Stöver and Rick Lines, 'Silence still = death: 25 years of HIV/AIDS in prisons', in *HIV/ AIDS in Europe: moving from death sentence to chronic disease management*, ed. by Srdan Matic, Jeffrey V. Lazarus, and Martin C. Donoghoe (Copenhagen: World Health Organization Europe, 2006), pp. 67–85.

5 Virginia Berridge, *AIDS in the UK: the making of policy, 1981–1994* (Oxford: Oxford University Press, 1996), pp. 220–1.

6 Examples include 'HIV/AIDS and US history', *Journal of American History*, 104.2 (2017), 431–60 (at 444); Catherine Cox and Hilary Marland, 'Broken minds and beaten bodies: cultures of harm and the management of mental illness in mid- to late nineteenth-century English and Irish prisons', *Social History of Medicine*, 31.4 (2018), 688–710; and the wider project 'Prisoners, Medical Care and Entitlement to Health in England and Ireland, 1850–2000': https://histprisonhealth. com (accessed 30 October 2019).

7 This impact is made plain in, for example, Don C. Des Jarlais, Samuel R. Friedman, and Jo L. Sotheran, 'The first city: HIV among intravenous drug users in New York City', in *AIDS: the making of a chronic disease*, ed. by Elizabeth Fee and Daniel M. Fox (Berkeley, CA: University of California Press, 1992), pp. 279–95; Karen Duke, *Drugs, prisons and policy-making* (London: Palgrave Macmillan, 2003); Gerry Stimson, 'Revising policy and practice: new ideas about the drugs problem', in *AIDS and drug misuse: the challenge for policy and practice in the 1990s*, ed. by John Strang and Gerry V. Stimson (London; New York: Routledge, 1990), pp. 121–31.

8 One such exception is an ACT UP protest at Pentonville Prison in London involving helium-filled condoms, which is mentioned in popular

accounts, including Simon Garfield, *The end of innocence: Britain in the time of AIDS* (London: Faber & Faber, 1995), pp. 181–2.
9 WHO, *Statement from the consultation on prevention and control of AIDS in prisons* (1987); Council of Europe, *Recommendation 1080*.
10 Global Programme on AIDS, *WHO guidelines on HIV infection and AIDS in prisons* (Geneva: World Health Organization, 1993). The Council of Europe also updated its guidelines that same year: Council of Europe, *Recommendation No. R(93)6 of the Council of Ministers* (Strasbourg: Council of Europe, 1993).
11 Council of Europe, *Draft report* (1988), appendix VII.
12 Timothy Harding and Georgette Schaller, *HIV/AIDS and prisons: updating and policy review: a survey covering 55 prison systems in 31 countries* (Geneva: WHO, 1992); Georgette Schaller and Timothy Harding, 'La Prévention Du SIDA Dans Les Prisons Européennes', *Sozial-Und Präventivmedizin*, 40 (1995), 298–301; Martin Moerings, 'AIDS in prisons in the Netherlands', in *AIDS in Prison*, ed. by Philip A. Thomas and Martin Moerings (Aldershot: Dartmouth, 1994), pp. 56–73 (at p. 59); 'Prison policies put inmates at risk', *British Medical Journal*, 310.6975 (1995), 278–83.
13 Claudio Mercandino, 'Carcere Di Torino L'Aids Uccide Ancora', *La Repubblica*, 25 February 1995.
14 Council of Europe, *Draft report* (1988), p. 8. For more on this way of conceptualising prisons and risk, see Janet Weston, 'Sites of sickness, sites of rights: HIV/AIDS, public health, and human rights in British prisons in the late twentieth century', *Cultural and Social History*, 16.2 (2019), 225–40.
15 Interview with Ben Hogg on *Today Tonight*, RTÉ, first broadcast 21 January 1986; interview with Roy Robertson and Carol Sutherland, Lothian Health Services Archive: https://media.ed.ac.uk/media/1_p2mympvw (accessed 30 October 2019); oral history interview with the founders of the Ana Liffey Drug Project, Frank Brady and Mara de Lacy, 17 November 2016. This and all subsequent oral history interviews cited here are available from the London School of Hygiene and Tropical Medicine Archive.
16 'Ban on movement at aids Scare gaol', *The Guardian*, 6 February 1985, p. 3.
17 Lill Scherdin, 'Aids in prisons in Norway', in *AIDS in Prison*, ed. by Philip A. Thomas and Martin Moerings (Aldershot: Dartmouth, 1994), pp. 7–19 (at p. 12).
18 John De Wit, 'AIDS in prisons in Belgium', in *AIDS in Prison*, ed. by Philip A. Thomas and Martin Moerings (Aldershot: Dartmouth, 1994), pp. 74–83 (at p. 80).

19 Janet Weston, 'Oral histories, public engagement, and the making of *Positive in Prison*', History Workshop Journal, 87 (2019), 211–33; Harding and Schaller, *HIV/AIDS and prisons*, p. 17.
20 Council of Europe, *Draft report* (1988), p. 9.
21 De Wit, 'AIDS in prisons in Belgium', p. 81; Council of Europe, *Report to the Irish government on the visit to Ireland carried out by the European Committee for the Prevention of Torture and Inhuman or Degrading Treatment or Punishment* (Strasbourg, 13 December 1995).
22 Council of Europe, *Report to the United Kingdom government on the visit to the United Kingdom carried out by the European Committee for the Prevention of Torture and Inhuman or Degrading Treatment or Punishment* (Strasbourg, 26 November 1991), p. 55; Council of Europe, *Report to the Norwegian government on the visit to Norway carried out by the European Committee for the Prevention of Torture and Inhuman or Degrading Treatment or Punishment* (Strasbourg, 21 September 1994), pp. 42–3; Scherdin, 'AIDS in prisons in Norway'.
23 Philip A. Thomas, 'AIDS in prisons in England & Wales', in *AIDS in Prison*, ed. by Philip A. Thomas and Martin Moerings (Aldershot: Dartmouth, 1994), pp. 20–9 (at p. 50). Council of Europe, *Draft report* (1988), appendix VIII.
24 Johannes Feest and Heino Stöver, 'AIDS in prisons in Germany', in *AIDS in Prison*, ed. by Philip A. Thomas and Martin Moerings (Aldershot: Dartmouth, 1994), pp. 20–9 (p. 23).
25 Council of Europe, *Draft report* (1988), appendix VIII.
26 Harding and Schaller, *HIV/AIDS and prisons*, p. 17. See also Harding's comments in *HIV infection and AIDS in the prison environment*, p. 199.
27 Schaller and Harding, 'La prévention du SIDA', p. 299.
28 James Freeman, 'Team wins award for plan to manage HIV prisoners', *Herald*, 13 February 1990.
29 Moerings, 'AIDS in prisons in the Netherlands', p. 67.
30 Schaller and Harding, 'La prévention du SIDA', p. 300.
31 Council of Europe, *Draft report* (1988), p. 9; Joachim Nelles, A. Fuhrer, H. P. Hirsbrunner, and Timothy Harding, 'Provision of syringes: the cutting edge of harm reduction in prison?', *British Medical Journal*, 317.7153 (1998), 270–3; Timothy Harding, 'AIDS in Prison', *The Lancet*, 330.8570 (1987), 1260–3.
32 Harding and Schaller, *HIV/AIDS and prisons*, p. 14.
33 Sally Perkins, *Access to condoms for prisoners in the European Union: final report* (London: National AIDS and Prisons Forum, 1998), p. 15.
34 Harding and Schaller, *HIV/AIDS and prisons*, table 3.1(c).
35 Perkins, *Access to condoms*, p. 14.

36 Janet Weston and Virginia Berridge, 'AIDS inside and out: HIV/AIDS and penal policy in Ireland and England & Wales in the 1980s and 1990s', *Social History of Medicine*, 33.1 (2020), 247–67.
37 *R v Secretary of State for Home Department Ex Parte Glen Fielding*, EWHC (Admin) 641 [1999]; 'Health victory for ex-prisoner in condom campaign', BBC News, 5 July 1999, available online at http://news.bbc.co.uk/1/hi/health/386301.stm (accessed 30 October 2019); Sue Quinn, 'Gay prisoners win access to condoms', *The Guardian*, 6 July 1999, available online at www.theguardian.com/uk/1999/jul/06/6 (accessed 4 November 2019); Jonathan Rayner, 'Elkan Abrahamson', *Law Gazette*, 4 November 2003, available online at www.lawgazette.co.uk/people/elkan-abrahamson/5038529.article (accessed 4 November 2019).
38 Harding and Schaller, *HIV/AIDS and prisons*, p. 15.
39 Nelles et al., 'Provision of syringes', p. 272.
40 Katie Stone and Sam Shirley-Beavan, *Global state of harm reduction 2018* (London: Harm Reduction International, 2018), p. 74.
41 Nelles et al., 'Provision of syringes', p. 270; Gen Sander, Alessio Scandurra, Anhelita Kamenska, Catherine MacNamara, Christina Kalpaki, Cristina Fernandez Bessa, Gemma Nicolás Laso, Grazia Parisi, Lorraine Varley, Marcin Wolny, Maria Moudatsou, Nuno Henrique Pontes, Patricia Mannix-McNamara, Sandro Libianchi, and Tzanetos Antypas, 'Overview of harm reduction in prisons in seven European countries', *Harm Reduction Journal*, 13.28 (2016), 3.
42 Avril Taylor, David Goldberg, John Emslie, John Wrench, Laurence Gruer, Sheila Cameron, James Black, Barbara Davis, James McGregor, Edward Follett, Janina Harvey, John Basson, and James McGavigan, 'Outbreak of HIV infection in a Scottish prison', *British Medical Journal*, 310.6975 (1995), 289; 'Prison policies put inmates at risk'.
43 LSHTM Health Promotion Research Unit, *Disinfecting tablets pilot project 1998: an evaluation* (London: LSHTM, 1999); Prison Reform Trust and National AIDS Trust, *HIV and hepatitis in UK prisons: addressing prisoners' healthcare needs* (London: Prison Reform Trust and National AIDS Trust, 2005), p. 12.
44 Joachim Nelles and Timothy Harding, 'Preventing HIV transmission in prison: a tale of medical disobedience and Swiss pragmatism', *The Lancet*, 346.8989 (1995), 1507–8.
45 Paola Bollini, Jean-Dominique Laporte, and Timothy Harding, 'HIV prevention in prisons: do international guidelines matter?', *The European Journal of Public Health*, 12.2 (2002), 83–9 (at 88); Stöver and Lines, 'Silence still = death'.

46 Geoffrey Dean, Aileen O'Hare, Aideen O'Connor, Michael Kelly, and Grainne Kelly, 'The opiate epidemic in Dublin 1979–1983', *Irish Medical Journal*, 78.4 (1985), 107–10; Fergus O'Kelly, 'Heroin abuse in an inner-city practice', *Irish Medical Journal*, 79.4 (1986), 85–7; John O'Connor, Sally Stafford-Johnson, Michael Kelly, and Gillian Byers, 'Attendance for drug misuse to Dublin accident and emergency departments', *Irish Medical Journal*, 79.11 (1986), 328–9.

47 Department of Health, *National Co-Ordinating Committee on Drug Abuse: first annual report* (Dublin: Stationery Office, 1986).

48 Dáil Éireann Ceisteanna – Questions: Drug Addiction in Prisons, 27 November 1985, Vol. 362 No. 2; 'Death in Mountjoy', *Today Tonight*, RTÉ, first broadcast 21 January 1986.

49 Interview with anonymous drug addiction worker in Dublin, 15 February 2017. See also Fiona Smyth, 'Cultural constraints on the delivery of HIV/AIDS prevention in Ireland', *Social Science and Medicine*, 46.6 (1998), 661–72.

50 Maurice Murphy, K. Gaffney, Owen Carey, Enda Dooley, and Fiona Mulcahy, 'The impact of HIV disease on an Irish prison population', *International Journal of STD and AIDS*, 3 (1992), 426–9.

51 Interview with Ben Hogg on *Today Tonight* (1986); interview with Frank Brady and Mara de Lacy; interview with former Mountjoy governor John Lonergan, 16 February 2017.

52 *Annual report on prisons and places of detention: 1986* (Dublin: Department of Justice, 1987), p. 7.

53 Dáil Éireann Private Notice Question: Death of Prisoner, 22 January 1986, Vol. 363 No. 1.

54 Interview with John Lonergan; interview with retired general practitioner Dr Fergus O'Kelly, 15 November 2016; interview with former probation and welfare officer Julian Pugh, 27 October 2016.

55 Dáil Éireann Written Answers – AIDS Test, 19 May 1987, Vol. 372 No. 10.

56 Interview with Frank Brady and Mara de Lacy; interview with John Lonergan; interview with Julian Pugh.

57 *Proceedings of the Conference of European National Sections: AIDS and human rights* (Geneva; Leiden: The International Commission of Jurists and the Netherlands Committee of Jurists for Human Rights, 1989), p. 37.

58 Criticisms became visible in, for example, Shane Butler and Marguerite Woods, 'Drugs, HIV and Ireland: responses to women in Dublin', in *AIDS: women, drugs, and social care*, ed. by Nicholas Dorn, Sheila Henderson, and Nigel South (London; Washington, DC: Falmer Press, 1992), pp. 51–69; Department of Health, *National AIDS Strategy*

HIV/AIDS in European prisons, 1980s–2000s   107

Committee: reports and recommendations of the Subcommittee on Care and Management of Persons with HIV/AIDS (Dublin: Stationery Office, 1992); *Report of the Advisory Committee on Communicable Diseases in Prison* (Dublin: Stationery Office, 1993); *Report to the Irish government on the visit to Ireland carried out by the European Committee for the Prevention of Torture and Inhuman or Degrading Treatment or Punishment* (Strasbourg: Council of Europe, 13 December 1995). See also interviews with John Lonergan and with former director of prison medical services Dr Enda Dooley, 16 February 2017.

59 Shane Butler and Paula Mayock, '"An Irish solution to an Irish problem": harm reduction and ambiguity in the drug policy of the Republic of Ireland', *International Journal of Drug Policy*, 16.6 (2005), 415–22; Shane Butler, 'The making of the methadone protocol: the Irish system?', *Drugs: Education, Prevention and Policy*, 9.4 (2002), 311–24.

60 Des Crowley, 'The Drug Detox Unit at Mountjoy Prison: a review', *Journal of Health Gain*, 3.3 (1999), 17–19.

61 Interview with Fergus O'Kelly; interview with anonymous addiction worker; interview with drug addiction worker Paul Hatton, 16 November 2016.

62 On this self-organisation, see Gemma Blok, 'The politics of intoxication: Dutch junkie unions' fight against the ideal of a drug free society, 1975–1990', in *The Transmission of Health Practices*, ed. by Martin Dinges and Roberts Jütte (Stuttgart: Franz Steiner Verlag, 2011), pp. 69–88.

63 Franz Trautmann, 'Peer support as a method of risk reduction in injecting drug-user communities: experiences in Dutch projects and the "European Peer Support Project"', *Journal of Drug Issues*, 25.3 (1995), 617–28 (at 621).

64 The following material draws on Trautmann, 'Peer support'; Heino Stöver and Franz Trautmann, 'The European Peer Support Project: Phase 3 – risk reduction activities in prisons', 1998, available online at www.bisdro.uni-bremen.de/Prisonfinal-report.htm (accessed 21 February 2017); Mary Cotter, *European Peer Support Seminar Dublin: a report* (Dublin, 1995).

65 Interview with anonymous drug addiction worker.

66 Interview with Julian Pugh; interview with anonymous addiction worker.

67 Oral history interview with general practitioner Dr Mel McEvoy, 15 February 2017.

68 Bollini, 'HIV prevention in prisons', p. 84.

69 'AIDS im Gefängnis', *Walliser Bote*, 3 October 1985, p. 3; 'Positif', *La Liberté*, 3 October 1985, p. 3; M. Zendali, 'Prisons: le virus dans la cellule', *La Liberté*, 6 June 1987, p. 39.
70 'Un cas de SIDA', *La Liberté*, 23 September 1985, p. 2.
71 'Aids im Gefängnis', *Thuner Tagblatt*, 21 December 1985, p. 9; 'Démission à Thorberg', *Le Nouvelliste*, 21 December 1985, p. 47.
72 'Un cas de SIDA', *La Liberté*, 23 September 1985, p. 2.
73 Harald K. H. Klingemann, 'Drug treatment in Switzerland: harm reduction, decentralization and community response', *Addiction*, 91.5 (1996), 723–36 (at 727). See also Joanne Csete and Peter J. Grob, 'Switzerland, HIV and the power of pragmatism: lessons for drug policy development', *International Journal of Drug Policy*, 23.1 (2012), 82–6.
74 Klingemann, 'Drug treatment in Switzerland'.
75 Nelles et al., 'Provision of syringes'.
76 Nelles and Harding, 'Preventing HIV transmission in prison'.
77 'Im Gefängnis Hindelbank gibt es ab April saubere Spritzen', *Thuner Tagblatt*, 31 January 1994, p. 3.
78 'Im Gefängnis Hindelbank'; Nelles and Harding, 'Preventing HIV transmission in prison'; Nelles et al., 'Provision of syringes'. See also the preface to *Harm reduction in prison: strategies against drugs, AIDS, and risk behaviour*, ed. by Joachim Nelles and Andreas Fuhrer (New York: Peter Lang, 1997) for a further account of the project's origins.
79 Nelles et al., 'Provision of syringes'.
80 'Automaten', *Freiburger Nachrichten*, 20 April 1999, p. 20.
81 Early criticism of this can be found in T. K. Whitaker, *Report of the Committee of Inquiry into the Penal System* (Dublin: Stationery Office, 1985).
82 Indeed, this is arguably how practices of methadone maintenance prescription were introduced to Irish prisons.
83 Interview with former head of nursing in the Irish Prison Service, Frances Nangle Connor, 15 November 2016.

4

Nursing a plague: nurses' perspectives on their work during the United Kingdom HIV/AIDS crisis, 1981–96

Tommy Dickinson, Nathan Appasamy, Lee P. Pritchard, and Laura Savidge

One evening shortly before Christmas 1984, David Ruffell began to feel 'very peculiar'. Walking around his local grocery store, he 'felt so ill [he] thought [he] was dying'. Thinking that he might have a venereal disease, he visited the Genito-Urinary Medicine Clinic in Hammersmith, London. The doctor at the clinic took one look at David and said, 'My God, you look absolutely awful', and immediately sent him for an X-ray. Upon reviewing the X-rays, he took hold of David's hand and told him, 'You're quite seriously ill. I'll be perfectly blunt: you've probably got a rare type of pneumonia called pneumocystis, which is connected with the AIDS problem. Until we can do a biopsy on your lung, we're going to admit you to Charing Cross Hospital immediately to treat you for that pneumonia.'[1]

At the hospital David waited alone behind curtains in the emergency department. No one would go near him. He shouted for a glass of water and a nurse responded by checking with the doctor first. She returned with the water but was wearing a mask and rubber gloves. David was eventually taken up to the ward and nurses placed him in isolation with a sign on the door that read 'Important: Barrier Nursing' and others saying 'Bio Hazard'. He was nursed in isolation for two weeks and 'never saw anybody unless they had a mask, gown and rubber gloves on'.[2] By Christmas 1987, three years after his initial diagnosis, David reported that he was 'very much alive'. He had taken up painting and was working on a series of pictures collectively entitled *Diagnosed AIDS*. To David, death from AIDS was 'a million miles away'. He did not have 'time to die. Bedsides, [he wanted] to learn how to play the steel drums next.' David Ruffell died on 5 July 1989. He was forty-nine years old.[3]

The United Kingdom's (UK) acute HIV/AIDS crisis emerged in 1981 and continued until 1996, when the evidence base for antiretroviral medication was confirmed and concepts of HIV/AIDS began to shift from untreatable terminal illness to manageable chronic disease.[4] By 1996, over 12,000 people had died from an AIDS-related illness in the UK. These years, before effective antiretroviral medication became widely available, were filled with suffering.[5] Many of those who delivered front-line care during this time were greatly affected by their experiences, the resonances of which linger on for them today. Their insightful and revealing memories deserve a prominent place in our accounts of the era.

This chapter draws on new oral histories of nurses who cared for people living with HIV/AIDS (PWHA), the loved ones of people who died of AIDS-related illnesses, and people who were diagnosed as HIV-positive between 1981 and 1996. Nurses working at the height of the HIV/AIDS crisis felt themselves to be fighting a 'plague', and to present their stories today is to illuminate a difficult time in the recent history of nursing. After describing our sources and reviewing the atmosphere surrounding HIV/AIDS in the UK in the 1980s, we explore the early difficulties and guidelines surrounding HIV/AIDS nursing in the UK. In describing the personal draw that HIV/AIDS care had for some nurses, particularly those who identified as 'queer',[6] we show how HIV/AIDS wards often became safe queer spaces, full of humour and campness. These spaces were welcomed by members of the queer community, but may have induced discomfort for some non-queer PWHA. We frame the work involved in nursing PWHA as 'dirty work', a term first coined by sociologist Everett C. Hughes.[7] Nurses undertaking this work were marred by their regular interactions with stigmatised individuals, and we discuss this in relation to Erving Goffman's concept of 'courtesy stigma', where those closely linked to people from stigmatised groups also acquire stigma.[8] Despite this – and perhaps sometimes because of it – many nurses worked to create a home-like environment on hospital wards for PWHA, and to craft new ways of caring that involved collaboration with 'experts by experience',[9] and a willingness to bend the rules. Nurses were faced with new kinds of decisions about what was permissible in these times of crisis. These experiences had a profound impact upon their lives, both professionally and personally.

Sources

Personal testimonials provide complex and nuanced accounts of HIV/AIDS, which can challenge 'sweeping or oversimplified cultural memories of this period' as a time only of extreme sadness, for example.[10] They also provide access to the experiences and views of hitherto marginalised individuals and communities, and can let us explore hidden or taboo subjects.[11] Historian John D'Emilo argues that these sources have the 'power to enrich, deepen and expand enormously' the history of sexuality,[12] and numerous scholars have similarly highlighted their value for suggesting new and nuanced histories of nursing.[13]

Face-to-face semi-structured oral history interviews were conducted by the lead author with twenty-two nurses who had cared for PWHA in various care settings across the UK, as well as seven loved ones of people who died of an AIDS-related illness, and four people who were diagnosed as HIV-positive in the 1980s. These interviews were audio-recorded and then transcribed, for ease of analysis and interpretation.[14] Participants were recruited via advertisements in the nursing press, the bulletins of HIV/AIDS organisations, and flyers advertising the project in sexual health clinics. Initial participants then put us in contact with other individuals. Participants were given a choice of where they would like to be interviewed, and most chose to be interviewed in their own home. In line with the views and practice of leading oral historian Penny Summerfield, all participants have been given pseudonyms here. As Summerfield has argued, this offers some protection for interviewees from the ultimate manifestation of the power inequity in the oral history relationship, namely, 'the historian's interpretation and reconstruction in the public form of print of intimate aspects of their lives'.[15]

There is a danger with this type of history, which pays close attention to individuals' attitudes and values regarding a sensitive issue, that interviewees and particularly the former nurses would tell us what they thought we wanted to hear. The fact that the interviews were conducted by a registered nurse (RN) may have helped to put former-nurse interviewees at ease and encouraged greater honesty, in that the interviewer was able to identify and empathise with elements of their story. He was in some respects an 'insider' in relation to the nurses he interviewed.[16] At the same time, there may have been elements of their practice that they did not feel able to reveal or admit to today, for fear that their past professional conduct would be judged in a negative way.

Summerfield argues that people do not simply remember what happened to them, but make sense of the subject matter by interpreting it through the contemporary language and concepts available to them. Therefore, the historian needs to understand not only the narrative offered, but also the meanings invested in it and their discursive origins.[17] Similarly, Simon Szreter and Kate Fisher note that personal testimonies are subjected to 'selection, omission, distortion and retrospection' and that these narratives are influenced with layers of 'cultural consciousness … communal conventions, idealisation and nostalgia'.[18] Nevertheless, they go on to argue that dialogue with the present should be seen as productive rather than distorting.[19] This is the approach we have adopted here, recognising that these interviews are not an exact representation of past events, but are in conversation with a present in which attitudes and ideas about HIV/AIDS have changed.

This project is based on testimonies from a small number of nurses who volunteered to be interviewed, most of whom had been working on specialist HIV wards. Thus, they are not representative of all nurses during the HIV/AIDS crisis. They are likely to be those who became particularly closely involved and invested in HIV work; other nurses will have had different experiences and behaved differently.

First encounters: nursing care of PWHAs, 1981–7

Community groups such as the London Lesbian and Gay Switchboard and the Terry Higgins Trust (THT) were mobilised by volunteers and led early piecemeal responses to the HIV/

AIDS crisis.[20] As discussed and described by historians including Virginia Berridge and Matt Cook, it was not until 1986 that the UK government became more robust and proactive in its reaction to this intensifying problem.[21] There emerged, as Berridge has described, a sense of wartime emergency.[22] That year, the secretary of state for health and social security, Norman Fowler, set up a cross-departmental unit to coordinate government attempts at 'crisis management'. Beginning in November 1986, and despite substantial Cabinet opposition and a distinct lack of enthusiasm from the Conservative prime minister, Margaret Thatcher, £20 million was spent on a major national public health campaign known by its tagline 'Don't Die of Ignorance'. This included television and billboard advertisements, and a leaflet posted to every household in the country.[23] In one television advert, a volcano erupted under a darkened sky and images of cascading rocks gave way to shots of a tombstone being chiselled, as the actor John Hurt gave a portentous voiceover.

> There is now a danger that has become a threat to us all. It is a deadly disease and there is no known cure. The virus can be passed during sexual intercourse with an infected person. Anyone can get it, man or woman. So far, it's been confined to small groups, but it's spreading, so protect yourself and read this leaflet when it arrives. If you ignore AIDS, it could be the death of you, so don't die of ignorance.[24]

As proliferating news reports about HIV/AIDS uncovered and fanned public alarm (and prejudice), the government's own campaign also drew on tactics of shock and fear. By the end of 1986, such highly emotive ways of communicating had become the norm in much public discourse about HIV/AIDS in the UK. Intermingled with this were anxieties about the supposed collapse of traditional homes and families, about race and immigration, and even about the long-promised nuclear apocalypse. These adverts aired only a few months after talks on reducing nuclear arms had collapsed at the Reykjavík Summit between Ronald Reagan and Mikhail Gorbachev, and a year after the Chernobyl nuclear power station disaster had given a glimpse of what nuclear fallout would mean for the world.[25] HIV/AIDS became, in one news headline, 'a moral Chernobyl':[26] one more disaster that the ills of the age seemed to have brought forth.

Internal government polling after the campaign revealed that 84 per cent of those asked felt confident that the campaign had educated them enough to avoid the risk of contracting HIV. In later years, this campaign would be hailed as a great success.[27] The UK government response to HIV/AIDS largely avoided the coercive measures that characterised, for example, official reactions in Sweden, Cuba, and the USA, including travel restrictions, forced disclosure, and quarantining.[28] Nevertheless, the broader context of fear was powerful and sustained. Some were uneasy about taking communion at church and chose to dip the wafer rather than drink directly from the cup. Others took their own scissors and combs to hairdressers. Flashpoints for fear included prisons, dentists, and blood transfusions, and hospitals in particular became a source of worry.[29]

Owing to the limited knowledge about routes of transmission, and the perceived risk of infection to other immune-compromised patients, PWHA admitted to National Health Service (NHS) hospitals were initially placed in isolation on general medical wards. This lack of knowledge, underscored by fear and ignorance, meant that patients were often poorly treated and subjected to theatrical shows of infection control, as recalled and described by Archibald Major. Archibald was an enrolled nurse on a surgical ward in 1983 and remembered a patient who came in with a breast abscess who was also living with AIDS. When the porters arrived to take him to theatre, 'they were completely gowned up. They had disposable trousers over their ordinary trousers; they'd got gowns on, three pairs of gloves, masks and visors.'[30] Walter Fredrick, whose partner died of an AIDS-related illness in 1984, remembered sitting with him in isolation: 'a hand would come round the door with food on it and it would just be dumped on the floor'.[31] Meanwhile, Christian Cowley recalled the 'repulsion and homophobia' that some physicians and nurses directed towards him and his partner, who died from an AIDS-related illness.[32]

As early as February 1985, professional nursing association and union the Royal College of Nursing (RCN) recognised that 'AIDS has highlighted serious deficiencies in the ability of some nurses to meet the psychosocial needs of their patients' and published a set of guidelines to remedy this entitled *The psychological support of the patient with AIDS*.[33] These guidelines acknowledged that caring for

PWHA would be challenging over the coming years, and that basic nurse education had, in most cases, failed to help nurses understand lifestyles different from their own. The guidelines stated that it was 'essential that nurses should be aware of their own feelings with regard to homosexuality, bi-sexuality or drug addiction before entering a situation where a patient may feel the need to discuss his life', since a nurse's 'initial and on-going attitudes may greatly affect the psychological outcome for these patients'. Nurses were encouraged to respect the personal and intimate relationships that PWHA had, and to be prepared to provide the person's significant other with the same information that they would normally only give an official next of kin. The RCN guidelines also emphasised that psychosocial care extended to include 'holistic' care, for not just the patient but also their loved ones. Nurses needed to provide emotional and psychological support to patients and their loved ones, from the moment of diagnosis through to palliative care and its related emotional difficulties. The guidelines explicitly stated that this 'care would need to be of a higher standard than previously seen due to the competing confidentiality issues and the emotionally charged nature of the diagnosis and concomitant work'.

Overall, this guidance placed a significant emphasis on the softer nursing skills that seemed necessary to care for this particular group. Christine Hallett has argued that responding to the emotions of patients and their loved ones is one of the 'arts' of nursing which have long been a central and unique aspect of nurses' work,[34] and many nurses later reflected on drawing upon these skills in the early days of HIV/AIDS. 'Suddenly here we were involved with the care of these critically ill patients, and nothing was working', remembered one interviewee. 'It felt like all we could do was make them comfortable and support their and their partner's emotions.'[35] Myrtle Cleator recalled the tension between official guidelines and providing the kind of care that felt necessary. With reference to a person in the final stages of AIDS, whom she had nursed in 1983, she noted that 'in those very early days the protocol was to "gown up" from head to toe every time you went into the room, even if you were just going in for a chat'. After giving her patient a bed bath and taking off her gloves, mask, and apron, she was about to leave the room when she noticed that he was crying. She 'walked over and gently wiped the tears from his eyes. I knew I should have put another pair of gloves on, but I just couldn't help myself.'[36] Recollections of difficult or emotional experiences such as these may have been disclosed as a result of the relationship of trust that was built up between the interview participants and the interviewer.[37] Conversely, though, this relationship could have been counterproductive in some cases, leaving individuals less willing to share memories that placed individuals or the nursing profession as a whole in a less positive light.

As hospitalisation and death rates rose, the NHS found itself ill-equipped to deal with the escalating crisis both organisationally and emotionally, as nursing student projects from that time indicate.[38] Responding to these emergent difficulties, the Charing Cross Hospital in London set up a Nursing Advisory Committee on the Care of Patients with AIDS in 1985, chaired by Robert Pratt, senior tutor of the hospital's School of Nursing. In April that year the committee published *AIDS: Towards a strategy of care*, which set out policy and procedure for nursing care of patients with HIV/AIDS at Charing Cross. The policy was evidently written in order to standardise the care of PWHA, and to quell anxieties among the Charing Cross care team. 'It is *not* necessary to put on aprons and gloves simply to go into the room to talk to the patient, take in a cup of tea or a meal tray', the policy stated. 'It is perfectly safe to touch patients without wearing gloves.' However, the policy still required PWHA to be nursed in isolation, with a 'Barrier Nursing' poster hung on the door, while the use of disposable utensils and crockery was also mandatory.[39] This no doubt derived from the belief, widespread at the time, that HIV could 'possibly be contracted by exposure to saliva'.[40]

The policy at Charing Cross emphasised the physical safety of staff and patients, and lacked discussion or guidance about how to meet the psychosocial needs of PWHA and their loved ones. Emanating from one hospital, it also indicated a paucity of national guidelines governing the care of PWHA at this time and the potential for great variation in levels of care between different hospitals around the country. Interviewees also noted regional variation; those who moved from rural locations to big cities like London and Manchester remembered receiving care from more dynamic, knowledgeable, and inclusive healthcare practitioners in urban centres.

'Looking after our own'

By the end of 1987, around 2,500 people were known to be HIV-positive in the UK, and over half of the 610 people known to have already died from AIDS-related illnesses had perished in this year alone. A significant step towards the professionalisation of the medical and nursing response to the crisis came with the widely publicised opening of Broderip Ward at London's Middlesex Hospital in April 1987: the first ward in the country dedicated to HIV/AIDS care. It was opened by Diana, Princess of Wales, who shook hands during the ceremony with nine patients without wearing protective clothing or gloves. In an interview with London newspaper the *Evening Standard*, an HIV-positive nurse who worked on the ward noted that this gave 'royal approval' to the fact that it was impossible to become infected through social contact.[41] Similar wards as well as community-based HIV/AIDS care services soon followed at sites across the UK in the late 1980s and early 1990s.

Within these services, nursing care began to change. This was partly to do with the increased knowledge and confidence signalled by the Princess of Wales' behaviour, but also flowed from those who worked there. Many of the nurses who elected to practice in these settings identified as queer and felt a sense of responsibility to their community, friends, and partners. Interviews suggested that support was forthcoming from across the queer community, with HIV/AIDS acting as a catalyst for this disparate and sometimes divided demographic to unite. Cecil Fenwick, whose partner died of an AIDS related illness in 1995, mused on this.

> The gay community changed, and we banded together. As opposed to being separate and polarised, and always looking out for sex. It was more like, 'we need to get together and look after each other.' If this guy from wherever doesn't have any family and he's sick, we need to support him: buy him groceries, wash his dishes. It became like watching out for your neighbours or your friends.[42]

Similarly, Cressida White, a nurse who identifies as a lesbian, reflected on her motivations for nursing those with HIV/AIDS at this time. 'I suppose it was about looking after our own', she said. 'It's peculiar really because, for whatever reason, it isn't common for gay men and lesbians to mix. It was like that before the onset of HIV and AIDS and it's like that again now really. But, during the 1980s and early 1990s, gay men and lesbians really came together. I think it drew out the caring nature of our community.'[43]

Others choosing to work in HIV/AIDS wards were heterosexual men and women whose loved ones had HIV/AIDS, or who simply perceived this as an exceptional health crisis to which they felt compelled to contribute their nursing skills. Some initially drifted into this area of practice through temporary agency shifts, but chose to work full-time in the field when they witnessed and experienced the dynamism and compassion of nursing care in this context. 'To jump into this body of nursing that was about respect, kindness, and gentleness towards these patients and their loved ones was just unbelievable, mind-blowing', one remembered.[44] Nurses also spoke about colleagues sometimes becoming patients; some nurses were HIV-positive themselves and were embraced by staff and patients alike in these environments. With a variety of motivations, these nurses created distinctive settings for delivering care and were at times symbols of continuity and compassion to their patients in rapidly changing and inauspicious times.

Many interviewees reflected on the high proportion of queer nurses who worked on HIV wards and the resultant humour and 'campness'.[45] Nurse Gertrude Fell, a trans woman, recalled that 'the ward was outrageous. The Charge Nurse used to have these gold lamé slippers that he would wear especially for the ward round.'[46] In her book *Dear Fatty*, comedian Dawn French described the HIV ward where a friend was nursed and died as 'the campest place in London', where there were 'nurses in drag and a cocktail trolley at 6pm'.[47] Meanwhile, Otto Best, who was diagnosed as HIV-positive in 1989, remembered 'a female nurse taking my blood and a male nurse in the corner doing whatever he was doing. She put the needle in, and I said, "Oh, you did that ever so well I shall have to give you a little prick award." To which the male nurse in the corner replied, "Nobody wants to win that, dear!"'[48] The queer humour that accompanied much HIV/AIDS nursing exemplifies Mary Douglas' account of jokes as 'a victorious tilting of uncontrol against control … the levelling of hierarchy, the triumph of intimacy over formality, of unofficial values over official ones'.[49] Removing hierarchies between nurse and patient, generating intimacy, and promoting new values were a key part of nursing on these wards.

Nurses and PWHA often spoke in their testimonies about the humour on these wards, emphasising that it was fun to be there despite the brutality of the condition. Participants were very keen to emphasise that this period 'wasn't all doom and gloom. There were as many laughs as there were tears.'[50] Although Farley Faragher, who was diagnosed as HIV-positive in 1985, 'felt like the Sword of Damocles was constantly hanging over my head', this necessarily changed the way he and many other HIV-affected people began to live their lives. He said, 'I realised that I only had a year or two more to live probably, so why not go out with a bang?'[51] 'You know', recalled Meredith Frampton, 'we had a lot of fun on the ward. There was a lot [of] mischief. We made it fun.'[52] Humour has also been recognised as a means by which healthcare workers rearrange their work, release tension, and create emotional alliances with their teams.[53] On HIV/AIDS wards, humour could release tension from the emotional labour of witnessing and coping with the atrocious daily realities of HIV/AIDS, and could create alliances between patients and nurses.

These alliances were also encouraged by a shared sense of community. Queer nurses described wanting to help because they felt that it was part of their duty to help others in their community. 'I just had to do something', said one. 'I couldn't sit back and watch as this vile syndrome wiped out my community.'[54] The proliferation of queer nurses requesting to work with PWHA saw many citing a preference to 'take care of their own'.[55] Others were drawn to the field of HIV/AIDS nursing because they knew how difficult it was to be queer at the time, with increased stigma for a perceived role in proliferating HIV/AIDS. Perhaps most infamously in this vein were the comments of James Anderson, the chief constable of Greater Manchester, who remarked in 1986 that homosexuals, drug addicts, and prostitutes who had HIV/AIDS were 'swirling in a human cesspit of their own making'.[56] There was an increase in hate crimes directed towards gay men and 'jokes' that took their association with AIDS for granted; GAY and AIDS became crude acronyms – 'got AIDS yet?' or 'arse-injected death sentence'.[57] Queer women were not immune from this; at the start of the HIV/AIDS crisis in the UK, lesbians were assumed in some quarters to be 'high-risk' as well, and some were barred from donating blood as a result.[58] Experiences of homophobia in public and in medical settings were one factor that encouraged many queer women to provide nursing care to those with HIV/AIDS.[59]

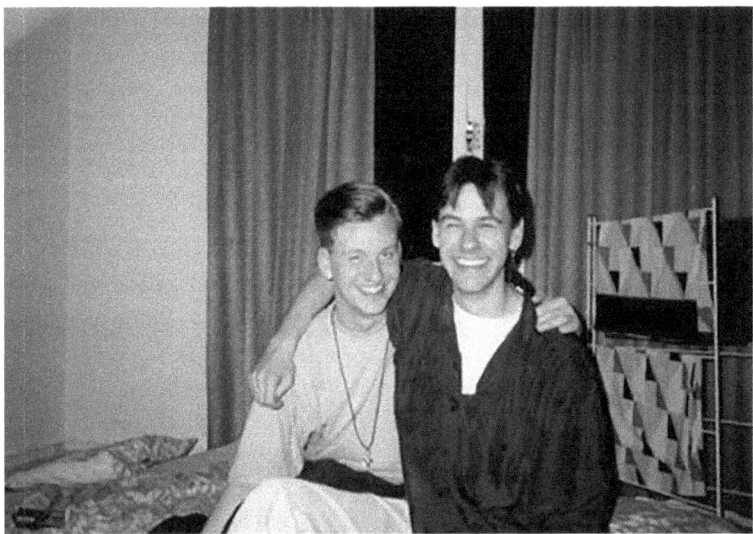

Figure 4.1 Sean Pert (left) and his friend Darren, taken when they lived together in Manchester, circa 1993/4. Darren died on 27 June 1996. He was twenty-seven years old.

PWHA and their loved ones spoke of the positive impact that queer nurses had on their care. When Sean Pert reflected on the nursing care his best friend Darren received (see Figure 4.1) before his death from an AIDS-related illness in 1996, he noted that 'Gay nurses were a godsend. I was just like, "Oh, thank god, we've got a gay nurse." There was a kind of unwritten understanding and compassion between us.'[60]

Although most patients on HIV/AIDS wards in the UK during this period were white, gay men, this was not the whole picture. Women consistently made up a minority of those diagnosed with HIV/AIDS, and towards the mid-1990s wards started to admit more Black people. In 1997, official statistics recorded over 400 Black individuals with AIDS in the UK; a majority of these were from 'presumed heterosexually acquired HIV infection'.[61] As described elsewhere in this collection, the epidemic also affected large numbers of injecting drug users, particularly in the cities of Liverpool, Edinburgh, and London. The experiences on the wards of those who did not identify as gay, who may have faced other forms of marginalisation or discrimination on the basis of gender, race, or drug use, have yet to be explored. As nurse George Jefferson reflected, 'I did occasionally think, would straight patients feel as comfortable in this environment as gay people? This was a small bit, but I was aware of it ... I understand why, up to a point', he concluded, 'because it's kind of reversing something that has been really awful for such a long time. We really want to make sure gay people are getting an amazing service and et cetera et cetera, but we also need to acknowledge there are a lot of straight people that are HIV-positive. Will they feel as comfortable in this environment? Most did', he thought, but 'some didn't'.[62]

Experts by experience and collaborative nursing

Against the often melodramatic backdrop of discussions or depictions of HIV/AIDS in the media in the 1980s, the relentless march of the disease emboldened some patients to self-organise, to speak up, and to speak out.[63] Virginia Berridge has analysed 'the rise of the patient' and the many HIV/AIDS activist organisations formed in the UK in the 1980s and 1990s, looking at patients gaining power through organisations set up to champion their cause.[64] These organisations were enormously influential in terms of shifting the power dynamics within medicine away from paternalism and towards collaboration. Here, we consider how this played out on the individual level, and its impact upon nursing.

Until the mid-1990s, HIV/AIDS was so devastating and puzzling that it was often those who had the most acute and personal lived experience with it, in the form of their own diagnoses, who were most knowledgeable. Patients were often as well-read and as up-to-date on treatment options and prognoses as their medical teams, meaning they sought recognition and collaboration with their nurses. Otto Best, who was diagnosed as HIV-positive in 1989, typifies this.

> A lot of us were young and we had awareness about what the ballgame was, and how fast things were moving. Many of our learning curves were almost the same as the nurses'. The style of nursing us was a shared relationship of a participating nature. You couldn't play the autocratic 'I'm the nurse, you're the patient' stuff, it didn't work. It was essentially a shared nursing experience.[65]

Moys Gillespie, a nurse who worked on an HIV/AIDS ward in the 1990s, reflected that she had learnt a great deal about HIV/AIDS treatments directly from PWHA, offering further confirmation of a newfound parity between nurses and patients; both groups stood together in the face of this crisis – not in abject, helpless suffering, but rather as equals at the cutting edge of medical advances. 'The guys taught you', Gillespie remembered. 'They knew their meds back to front. You'd take the drug trolley around (and there'd be lots and lots), but the guys would say to you "I need that and that." That was my first example of patients taking control of their own health in terms of questioning. It took a little bit of getting used to, but I thought it was amazing.'[66] This level of knowledge and ability among some PWHA to express their concerns and choices fed into the shaping of the care environment. Elias Pound, who was diagnosed as HIV-positive in 1988, describes this characteristic from his point of view: 'We were not a group of people who said, "Oh, would you please give us better care?" We demanded it!'[67] Aloysius Murphy used the same phrasing, remembering in positive terms the distinctive environment on the HIV/AIDS ward in which his partner had received care and the quality of nursing, adding that 'I think the patients demanded this'.[68]

The rise of the expert by experience was arguably connected to a broader rhetoric of personal empowerment, developed from challenges to medical paternalism which began in the 1960s. The anti-psychiatry movement, for example, or the broader critique of medicine laid down in Ivan Illich's (in)famous 1974 book *Medical nemesis*, sought to challenge and disrupt the power of the medical professional and the medical establishment.[69] The phenomenon of the expert by experience HIV/AIDS patient also had antecedents in the fight for gay rights of the 1970s. Fights for gay rights, anti-psychiatry, and challenges to medical authority all involved activism, and activism of course plays a large role in histories of HIV/AIDS. In the context of nursing, we see not just an expert patient but an activist patient.

This was not the grand-scale HIV/AIDS activism we may expect but, rather, small-scale efforts to change knowledge, attitudes, and norms by influencing and teaching healthcare practitioners so that the experiences of PWHA in the future would be better. Elizabeth

Quayle, who had nursed PWHA in a hospice, expressed this idea and reflected on the PWHA that she nursed, offering her own interpretation for the genesis of the activist patient and the daily struggle they faced on the ward.

> These people were really up against it. I also think that they were used to 'bucking the norm', so they've been used to pushing against establishment ... That's what came across to me, and they were now very confident in doing that ... So, there was a lot of 'we don't do that. We don't like that.' And you could feel the challenge in their eyes.[70]

Some patients therefore sought and captured power within their healthcare experiences, through a combination of expert knowledge and an ability to challenge medical authority and to demand a certain quality of life in hospital.[71] Nurses also had to be willing to learn from their patients. Shortly after starting on an HIV/AIDS ward, Marie Kelly recalled sitting on the bed of a patient who had been newly diagnosed with AIDS. He was telling her about all the different types of sex he had and asking about the risks involved. 'I felt so naïve', Marie said. 'I'd never even heard of "S&M", let alone what it entailed! I remember thinking "I've got a lot to learn!"'[72] Where patients could express themselves and nurses were prepared to listen and learn, care could become more collaborative.

This experience was far from universal. PWHA in prisons, for one, did not have the same sense of agency. Prisons often exacerbated the concerns of PWHA that not enough was being done to help them. John Campbell felt that he knew more than his 'nurses' in prison, having correctly identified that most were not RNs but correctional officers with six weeks of medical training.[73] An internal report quoted people in prison stating that the prison doctor 'frightens me because he gives me such poor explanations of what's going on', or that the medical advice received about HIV/AIDS in prison always contradicted that of the THT, leaving PWHA extremely worried.[74] PWHA in prison were aware that they were sequestered from the NHS, from RNs, from developing medical knowledge about HIV/AIDS, and from voluntary organisations like the THT; they were one example of PWHA whose circumstances severely compromised their ability to become experts, and who did not experience the collaborative care that was praised elsewhere.

Nursing and 'dirty work'

Nurses often reflected on the strain of the labour involved in nursing PWHA. All the nurses that we interviewed spoke of the intensive physiological and psychological nursing care that was required, and the difficulties that this entailed. Everett Hughes first coined the term 'dirty work' in 1951 and developed it further in 1958; he used it to conceptualise occupations considered socially, morally, or physically degrading or disgusting.[75] Nurse and researcher Catherine Prebble, in her discussion of psychiatric nursing as 'dirty work', has clarified that these occupations are not inherently dirty, but rather they carry an idea of 'dirtiness'.[76] Members of a group who carry out 'dirty work' come to personify the work itself, and therefore become 'dirty workers'.[77]

This can usefully be applied to nursing PWHA. Physically, nurses for PWHA were intimately involved with the often unpleasant aspects of bodily function: elimination, pain, washing, and handfeeding. Annie Crebin recalled how 'thin and frail' the PWHA that she nursed in the 1980s and 1990s were: 'young men were literally skin and bones in bed. We had to turn them regularly to stop pressure sores, but each turn caused them excruciating pain.'[78] Patients' beds would often need changing up to five or six times a night because of night sweats or cryptosporidium diarrhoea. Freda Rutter remembered this in vivid detail, saying that there 'was literally litres and litres of brown water pouring out of these people. And the night sweats; it was like you'd poured a bucket of water onto their bed. They were sopping.'[79] Many had difficulty eating and drinking owing to oesophageal candidiasis, which was 'literally coming out of their mouths and round their face'.[80]

Socially, nurses were also marred by their regular interactions with these stigmatised individuals, described by Erving Goffman as 'courtesy stigma'.[81] Nurses for PWHA were expected to provide succour and care for a highly stigmatised group, experiencing severe psychological and physiological distress – a duty that society demanded, but also reviled. A poignant example of courtesy stigma was that many nurses decided to keep their place of work confidential from friends and family, believing that it could give rise to panic, suspicion, and unwanted questioning. Indeed, when Martha Munro told her father that she was going to work on an HIV/AIDS ward he was unequivocal in his condemnation of her choice, asking 'Why the hell would you put yourself at risk for a bunch of queers? It's their own fault they've got this disease – it serves 'em right – let 'em rot I say!'[82]

Some nurses encountered hostility from other hospital staff,[83] creating a sense of segregation. Bertha Brown recalled feeling isolated from and stigmatised by colleagues in other departments of the hospital. 'I can remember being in the canteen with colleagues from the HIV ward, and getting a sense of people looking and not wanting to sit with us.'[84] Sarah Shimmon shared a similar memory, saying that 'I felt we were completely isolated and didn't really mix with other people much in hospital. There was a sense we were slightly apart.'[85] Consequently, many nurses reported that the HIV/AIDS wards where they worked had less surveillance compared to other wards within the hospital. 'We were pretty much left to our own devices', remembered one. 'People were scared to come onto the ward, so they just left us to it.'[86] As the next section discusses, this independence from mainstream hospital oversight and activity was not without some advantages.

Testing boundaries and 'care-crafting'

The stigma that was attached to HIV/AIDS care providers fostered environments where nurses, often free from direct managerial oversight, could dictate care and shift boundaries with much greater ease. Nurses recounted the ways in which the type of care they provided on HIV/AIDS wards was different from that which they had provided in other care settings. Nurses described watching out for the nurse administrator while patients smoked forbidden cigarettes or when pets were brought onto the ward to comfort their dying companion. Couples would lie in bed together behind closed doors or curtains, with no questions asked as to the extent of their intimacy. One nurse took a patient for a ride on the back of a motorbike a few days before the patient died, because it was something that the patient had always wanted to do. Other nurses discreetly palmed clean needles for intravenous drug users.[87] In this way, nurses collaborated in different ways with their patients, creating new kinds of nursing environments and care. For some, this work was itself a form of activism. 'We took a stand', remembered one interviewee: 'we were activists at a time when support from our leaders and colleagues was mainly absent'.[88]

Nurses remembered becoming aware of the necessity for these environments to be inclusive and welcoming. Jane Bruton had been the sister on an HIV/AIDS ward and spoke of creating a home-like environment that was 'a place of warmth, safety and love'.[89] Marsha Bausch similarly reflected on the contrast between the HIV/AIDS ward she worked on and other wards in the hospital.

> At one point the ward had to move to another ward because they were going to repaint it. They split the ward in half and the other half was a surgical ward, which was run by somebody who'd been in the army – a military charge nurse. The patients were woken up at 6am – full blaring lights went on, drugs were given out and people were left standing 'white and wobbly'. We just had a curtain separating the two halves of the ward. So, in our half of the ward, it would be dark and peaceful, and there might be some sort of earth music playing, with scented candles and aromatherapy. As the patients woke up one by one, we would individually offer them breakfast. We'd make them toast or cornflakes, whatever they wanted. We'd always wait for them to wake up. We'd make sure that they had their drugs, but then let them go back to sleep, if they wanted. It was so marked, the contrast between the wards.[90]

Aloysius Murphy, whose partner died from an AIDS-related illness in 1987, agreed that the HIV/AIDS ward where his partner was nursed and died was 'unlike any other ward. It had an amazing energy, strength, and vitality. Nurses were liberal and vibrant in their care.'[91]

As we analysed and interpreted these testimonies, it became apparent that there were times when these memories were more important as an indication of personal development and meaning than as a source of empirical data. Peter Pain, for example, when recalling his time working on the HIV/AIDS ward, stated that 'it was a special chapter of my life … as I reflect on that time, I always remember the blazing sun streaming through the big windows on the ward and how bright and beaming it made the ward look'.[92] His memory of sunny weather was not a factual account of endless sunshine, but a way of conveying his happy memories of the time spent working on this ward. This offers a way to understand the subjective experiences shared in interviews and the numerous constructed identities that they connote, especially in relation to the meanings that these nurses later placed on their work caring for PWHA. Indeed, Elizabeth Kennedy argues that to supplement the authenticity of the data, historians must learn in this way from the subjective nature of oral history interviews.[93]

Being liberal and vibrant, as already indicated, could mean breaking the rules – or, rather, creating new ones for this unprecedented situation. This required thinking beyond standard training and policy. Paaie Clague explained that nurses on HIV/AIDS wards 'had to be really imaginative in our care and work outside the box. On many occasions, this meant we broke the "rules", which was brilliant. That said, looking back, there were no rules; we didn't have rules because we didn't know what the rules were. We'd never done it before.' The guiding principle in this context was

> being human with people, not just being the Nurse. Sometimes we made unorthodox and, on reflection, quite bold clinical judgements and decisions, which nurses on other wards would have probably baulked at. That makes it sound like it was unprofessional; it wasn't – there was a great deal professionalism. We just did just whatever we could to enhance their stay and reduce their fear and suffering. And I can honestly say that every decision we made felt completely like it was the right thing to do.[94]

Paaie's testimony suggests that the care of PWHA necessitated new ways of thinking, requiring imagination and confidence. It also required self-reflection and a willingness to question; as Margaret Kidd remembered, '[e]very decision you made you looked at and asked why'.[95]

The particularities of HIV/AIDS also meant that nurses had to navigate new and challenging formulations of medical ethics regarding confidentiality. Breaches of confidentiality could include indirect disclosures of an HIV/AIDS diagnosis; for example, a patient's cadaver wrapped in a body bag would indicate that they had died of an AIDS-related illness, as other deceased patients were not subjected to such robust infection-control measures. There was the worry of a 'double coming-out', since for a man to reveal to friends and family that he had HIV/AIDS would also imply or confirm that he was homosexual. HIV-related stigma was also present within communities that were marginalised on the basis of sexuality or race and ethnicity, and revealing an HIV diagnosis could prompt ostracisation and isolation.⁹⁶ On the specialist HIV/AIDS ward in Edinburgh, where HIV/AIDS was prevalent among those injecting drugs, Elizabeth Quayle recalled that nurses had to be mindful of keeping patients' identities secret in case they were known to one another through drug debts, which could lead to violence on the ward.⁹⁷

Hugo Pearl, an RN in charge of an HIV/AIDS ward in the early 1990s, described in detail one example of the decision-making that nurses engaged in, across often undesignated ethical terrain. His story is worth quoting in full.

> This patient comes around the corner from his bed. And he's dressed head-to-toe in leather, carrying a little leather cap. I said, 'And where the hell are you going?' It was like ten o'clock at night. He said, 'I just thought I'd pop out for a drink.' I went, 'Sweet cheeks, I've got a list of medication as long as my arm to get through you. You know what you're like, it'll be an eight-hour thing.' He said, 'I just wanted to go out for a quick drink, I'm sick of being cooped up in here.' And I went, 'I want you back in here in an hour, all right? Where are you going?' He told me where he was going, I can't remember what club or pub, or wherever he was going. And off he trots. I told no one he had left. He signed no release forms, nothing! He was just, 'Thanks love!' and off he trotted. At about one or two in the morning, I get a call from the front hall who said: 'I've got a couple of fellas down here and one of them says he's a patient on your ward.' I thought: 'Oh thank God he's back. Someone's obviously brought him back.' And so, I said to the guy on the phone: 'All right, just send him up.' So, he walks down the ward, it's pitch-black. He's still dressed in leather, chaps, you know, the whole box and dice. He leaned up against the nursing station as pissed as a rat, and he said to me: 'Can my friend stay?' And I said: 'It's not a bloody hostel, dolly. It's a hospital with beds, they're all single.' And he said: 'Aw, he's missed his last bus.' I looked up the top of the ward and there's this guy stood there smiling like a Cheshire cat. He said, 'He can't sleep in the street.' And I thought 'well, that just beggars belief. I'm sorry, you go out, you're a patient on a HIV unit, and you pick up some trade and bring 'em back.' So, I said: 'All right, he can stay.' So, we pulled the curtains round, got him into bed, and you know, the other guy got into bed as well. And I said 'If I hear anything going on behind this screen then I'll be in here every five minutes. This drip better not be stopped

either!' And I plugged that in and I said: 'You, smart ass, you will be out of this ward by 6:30 when the buses start because when the day staff come in and find what's going on, I'm for the chop, not you, all right? So, don't mess with me, do as you're told!' Anyway, I don't know what went on in there, but sure enough he'd left by 6:30.[98]

There is a knowingness in the telling of this riotous yarn; it is funny and presents itself like a kind of queer pantomime, with closed curtains, costumes, and Hugo's reprimands and threats to burst in on the pair, even though he was clearly a fairly willing accomplice. It depicts a hospital ward unlike most others, in which patients' wishes were respected no matter how unconventional, and where humour was never far away.

While Hugo's clinical judgement and decision-making lay beyond the boundaries of what would have been deemed acceptable by professional codes of conduct (then or now), his actions on that night enabled a one-night stand to blossom into a loving relationship. The visitor who had missed his bus became the patient's boyfriend, and was with him by his side until he died. Hugo was care-crafting to allow his patient to retain a quality of life that he had lost, not just because of the psychological and physiological effects of the disease, but also because of the 'social death' that followed. Social death saw many who were already in an out-group shunned by society, struggling to remain connected to a community.[99] Letting a patient leave the ward on that night allowed a man living with AIDS a rare moment of re-entry into a social realm that had seemed off-limits.

Previous research has categorised rule-breaking and subterfuge on the part of nurses as 'responsible subversion'.[100] Our findings complement but complicate this, spotlighting the emotional component to this in the case of HIV/AIDS. The Denver Principles, written in 1983 by AIDS activities in the USA to help guide the care and treatment of PWHA, advocated that healthcare professionals should 'get in touch with their feelings (e.g., fears, anxieties, hopes, etc.) about AIDS and not simply deal with AIDS intellectually'.[101] For many nurses, these feelings were complex; as discussed above, many were drawn to working on HIV/AIDS wards for very personal reasons. Deeply felt emotions mediated the everyday lives of many gay men, including gay nurses such as Hugo, during the HIV/AIDS crisis. This is evident in the personal testimonials from

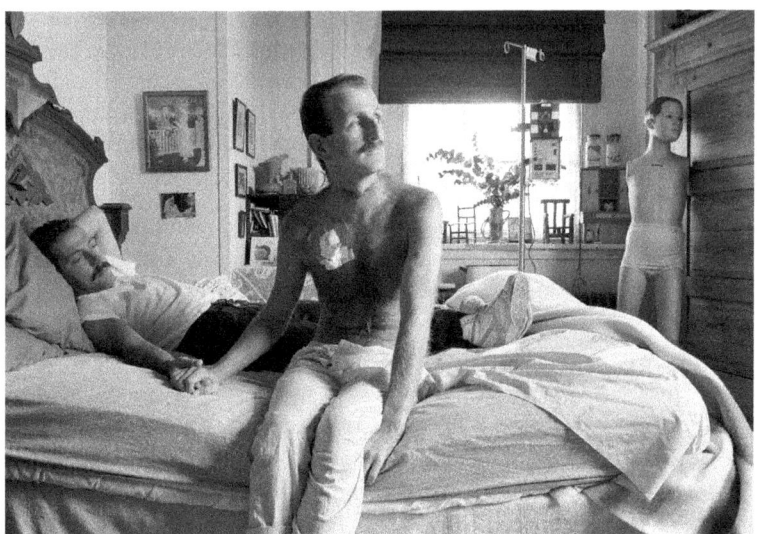

Figure 4.2 David (lying down) and Eric (sitting) at their home in Boston, MA, 1986. Photograph reprinted with permission by Sage Sohier from her series 'At Home with Themselves: Same-Sex Couples in 1980s America'.

the USA; David, photographed with his partner Eric in Figure 4.2, recalled that he 'hated everyone when [he] found out his [partner] Eric had AIDS, including Eric. I mean, I was angry at him for getting this disease. Angry at myself for being gay, angry for having those feelings of anger.'[102] Luc Ferrier, a nurse who worked on an HIV/AIDS ward in the 1990s and who is also an HIV-positive gay man, described how his social life centred on attending the wakes of friends who had died, where he 'cried and cried until I thought I couldn't cry anymore, then I cried some more'.[103] Matt Cook has explored emotions in the British context, finding that many gay men felt they had to hide the grief, anger, frustration, anxiety, and shame experienced in the context of 'serial loss and anti-gay backlash trading in blame and fear'.[104] Hugo's responsible subversion may well have been a reaction to this, in that it allowed grief and frustration to be set aside in favour of humour and defiance. This subversion became a celebration of queer joy and virility in the face of death.

Conclusion

The unique nature of the nursing work involved in caring for PWHA in the 1980s and 1990s had a lasting impact on the nurses that we interviewed. Many said that it had transformed them, not only professionally but also personally. For many of the nurses we interviewed, these memories were so powerful that they reportedly felt like they had occurred only moments ago. Nurses reported that they were still in contact with their colleagues from those years, and that the strong emotional bonds with their peers that developed had not diminished. The impact of this work was treasured, and the period was understood as a time of intense joy and intense sadness, of humanity experienced to the fullest, stripped of façade and pretence. Nurse Hattie Price became emotional as she reflected on what it meant to her to remember this aspect of her nursing career.

> It was a special part of my life. It sounds odd, but some of the most joyful memories I have are working on [the HIV/AIDS] ward. It made me who I am now, and it taught me how to be a brilliant nurse. It changed my view on the world, particularly working in an environment that I was the minority, the other [becoming emotional]. It was a ridiculously amazing experience that defined the rest of my life.[105]

This chapter contributes to the history of nursing in the UK by highlighting these experiences during the HIV/AIDS crisis of the 1980s and early 1990s, and the ways in which the care of individuals belonging to stigmatised groups was crafted. It reveals the personal draw that HIV/AIDS care had for some, particularly for nurses who identified as queer, and the distinctive nursing environment that was created, in which humour played a prominent role. It also adds to our understanding of the emergence of the expert by experience; assertive PWHA became experts and took control of their own care, prompting nurses to collaborate with them. In this context, nurses made bold decisions about what actions were permissible in times of crisis.

Nurses caring for PWHA in the 1980s and early 1990s worked through a long and difficult period, when there were limited biomedical solutions on hand. The unpredictable physical, psychological, and social harms inflicted by HIV/AIDS threatened to overwhelm life on the wards, and placed a heavy burden on nursing professionals who themselves suffered 'courtesy stigma' and had to grapple with complex emotions. In this most difficult of moments, nurses found richness in their work with PWHA by drawing on their 'artistic' nursing skills to craft the best care possible. Displaying compassion, creativity, and fortitude, many nurses in the UK joined forces with their patients to forge ahead with collaborative care, and deserve a place in HIV/AIDS history.

Acknowledgements

The authors would like to thank the Barbara Brodie Nursing History Fellowship, the Royal College of Nursing Monica Baly Bursary, the Wellcome Trust, and the King's College London Undergraduate Research Fellowship for funding the project on which this chapter is based, and Professors Barbara Mann-Wall, Matt Cook, and Kenneth White for their incisive comments on previous drafts of the chapter. Dr Dickinson would like to give thanks to the School of Nursing at the University of Virginia, USA for allowing him the time to work on this project during his time there as Talbott Visiting Professor of Nursing. Finally, we owe a unique debt to the participants who were interviewed as part of the project. Some of their testimonies were quite difficult to hear and we admire their bravery in retelling their stories.

Notes

1. David Ruffell, *Walking after midnight: gay men's life stories* (London: Routledge, 1989), pp. 95–108.
2. *Ibid.*, p. 102.
3. *Ibid.*, p. 109.
4. See, for example, Matt Cook, 'AIDS, mass observation and the fate of the permissive turn', *Journal of the History of Sexuality*, 26 (2017), 239–72; Simon Garfield, *The end of innocence: Britain in the time of AIDS* (London: Faber & Faber, 1994).
5. See, for example, Colin Clews, *Gay in the 80s: from fighting for our rights to fighting for our lives* (London: Troubador Publishing, 2017); Craig Hanlon-Smith, 'His story, her story, it's all our stories', *GSCENE Gay Magazine*, 7 January 2016, p. 37.

6 We have used the term 'queer' in this chapter to reflect queer in its broadest sense, not to collapse people together, but to mean those considered queer in whatever (gendered or sexualised) ways.
7 Everett C. Hughes, *Men and their work* (Glencoe, CA: Forgotten Books, 1958); Everett C. Hughes, 'Work and the self', *Social psychology at the crossroads*, ed. by John H. Rohrer and Muzafer Sherif (New York: Books for Libraries Press, 1951), pp. 313–23.
8 The phrase 'courtesy stigma' was used by Erving Goffman in *Stigma: notes on the management of spoiled identity* (Harmondsworth: Touchstone Press, 1963).
9 An expert by experience (EbE) is someone who is able to articulate lessons and suggestions from their own 'lived' experience of health challenges. Their expertise is based on their own individual experiences, enabling them to speak with authenticity. EbEs can also be in a unique position to connect to others with similar experiences, bringing a wider range of 'lived' experience views to partnership working.
10 Matt Cook, ' "Archives of feeling": the AIDS crisis in Britain 1987', *History Workshop Journal*, 83 (2017), 57.
11 See, for example, Tommy Dickinson, *'Curing queers': mental nurses and their patients, 1935–74* (Manchester: Manchester University Press, 2015).
12 John D'Emilio, 'Afterword: if I knew then…', in *Bodies of evidence: the practice of queer oral history*, ed. by Nan A. Boyd and Horacio N. Roque Ramirez (Oxford: Oxford University Press, 2012), p. 269.
13 See, for example, Geertje Boschma, 'Community mental health nursing in Alberta, Canada: an oral history', *Nursing History Review*, 20 (2012), 103–35; Jane Brooks, *Negotiating nursing: British Army sisters and soldiers in the Second World War* (Manchester: Manchester University Press, 2018); Peter Nolan, 'Psychiatric nursing past and present: the nurses' viewpoint' (PhD dissertation, University of Bath, 1989).
14 Anna Green, 'Unpacking the stories', in *Remembering: writing oral history*, ed. by Anna Green and Megan Hutching (Auckland: Auckland University Press, 2004), p. 11.
15 Penny Summerfield, *Reconstructing women's wartime lives* (Manchester: Manchester University Press, 1998), p. 27.
16 Catherine Prebble, a registered mental health nurse, believed she was an 'insider' when interviewing mental health nurses, mainly due to perceptions of a shared stigma by association with mental illness and shared insight into feeling misunderstood by other nurses and by the public. Catherine M. Prebble, 'Ordinary men and uncommon women: a history of psychiatric nursing in New Zealand public mental

hospitals, 1939–1972' (PhD dissertation, University of Auckland, 2007), p. 23.
17 Penny Summerfield, 'Culture and composure: creating narratives of the gendered self in oral history interviews', *Cultural and Social History*, 1 (2004), 69.
18 Simon Szreter and Kate Fisher, *Sex before the sexual revolution: intimate life in England, 1918–1963* (Cambridge: Cambridge University Press, 2010), p. 51.
19 *Ibid.*, p. 11.
20 The Terry (now Terrence) Higgins Trust is a UK charity that campaigns on and provides services relating to HIV/AIDS and sexual health. It was established in 1982 and was the first British charity to support people living with HIV/AIDS.
21 Virginia Berridge, *AIDS in the UK: the making of policy 1981–1994* (Oxford: Oxford University Press, 1996); Cook, 'Archives of feeling'. See also Garfield, *The end of innocence* ; Norman Fowler, *AIDS: don't die of prejudice* (London: Biteback Publishing Ltd, 2014).
22 Berridge, *AIDS in the UK*, pp. 6–7.
23 See Chapter 2 in this volume for a detailed analysis of the television advert and leaflet that circulated in Italy at around the same time, and Chapter 5 for the alternative route followed in Wales.
24 These public information films are available online at the British Film Institute's YouTube channel: www.youtube.com/watch?v=yVggWZuFApI and www.youtube.com/watch?v=iroty5zwOVw (accessed 25 October 2021).
25 Nuclear dangers were thoroughly etched into public consciousness; films such as *Threads* (1984) memorably depicted the extreme medical, economic, social, and environmental consequences of nuclear war on the city of Sheffield in northern England. *Threads* (dir. Mick Jackson; London: British Broadcasting Corporation, Nine Network, 1984), DVD; *The 80s with Dominic Sandbrook* (dir. Alex Leith; London: British Broadcasting Corporation, 2017), DVD; Cook, 'Archives of feeling', p. 57.
26 Quoted in Cook, 'Archives of feeling', p. 60.
27 Fowler, *AIDS: Don't die of prejudice*, p. 27; Jon Kelly, 'HIV/AIDS: why were the campaigns successful in the West?' *British Broadcasting Corporation News Magazine*, 28 November 2011, p. 6.
28 Steve Connor and Sharon Kingman, *The search for the virus* (Harmondsworth: Penguin, 1989), pp. 6–11; Matt Cook, 'AIDS, mass observation, and the fate of the permissive turn', *Journal of the History of Sexuality*, 26.2 (2017), 244.

29 Berridge, *AIDS in the UK*; George Severs, 'The Church of England's response to the HIV/AIDS epidemic, c. 1982–2000' (master's thesis, University of Cambridge, 2017); Cook, 'Archives of feeling', p. 61.
30 Interview with Archibald Major, 22 February 2017.
31 Interview with Walter Fredrick, 18 April 2017.
32 Interview with Christian Cowley, 13 April 2017.
33 Royal College of Nursing, *The psychological support of the patient with AIDS* (February 1985). The RCN was also active in lobbying Parliament to pass an official declaration of the rights of people with HIV/AIDS in 1992. See Royal College of Nursing Archive (Edinburgh), *The Royal College of Nursing Council minutes: The UK declaration of the rights of people with HIV & AIDS* (RCN 20.2–3), February 1992.
34 Christine E. Hallett, 'Nursing: the lost art?', lecture at the University of Tromsø. Available online at https://mediasite.uit.no/Mediasite/Play/152d249a450941f9bf6b770cf9ba30581d (accessed 25 October 2021).
35 Interview with Polly O'Sullivan, 26 April 2017.
36 Interview with Myrtle Cleator, 8 August 2017.
37 See, for example, Szreter and Fisher, *Sex before the sexual revolution*, p. 6.
38 See, for example, Fiona Huntsman, 'An aid for AIDS' (final-year project, Middlesex Hospital School of Nursing, 1984); Elizabeth A. Cave, 'Equipped to care? Awareness of AIDS and HIV amongst student nurses' (final-year project, Middlesex Hospital School of Nursing, 1985).
39 Robert J. Pratt, *AIDS: towards a strategy of care* (London: Charing Cross Hospital Nursing Advisory Committee on the Care of Patients with AIDS, 1985). Emphasis in original.
40 Huntsman, 'An aid for AIDS', p. 60.
41 Quoted in Garfield, *The end of innocence*, p. 280.
42 Interview with Cecil Fenwick, 7 April 2017.
43 Interview with Cressida White, 4 August 2017.
44 Interview with Meredith Frampton, 13 February 2017.
45 Campness is used here to mean 'a characteristically gay way of handling the products of a culture through irony, exaggeration, trivialization, theatricalization and an ambivalent making fun out of the serious and respectable'. Richard Dyer, *The culture of queers* (London: Bloomsbury Publishing, 2002), p. 250.
46 Gertrude Fell, interviewed 26 January 2017.
47 Dawn French, *Dear Fatty* (London: Random House, 2009), p. 347.

48 Interview with Otto Best, 26 April 2017.
49 Mary Douglas, *Implicit meanings: selected essays in anthropology*, 2nd edn (London: Routledge, 1999). See also Hannah J. Elizabeth, '*Love carefully* and without "over-bearing fears": the persuasive power of authenticity in late 1980s British AIDS education material for adolescents', *Social History of Medicine*, 34.4 (2021), 1317–42.
50 Interview with Ethel Caine, 6 September 2017.
51 Interview with Farley Faragher, 22 March 2017.
52 Interview with Meredith Frampton, 13 February 2017.
53 Carmen Moran and Margaret Massam, 'An evaluation of humour in emergency work', *The Australian Journal of Disaster and Trauma Studies*, 3 (1997), 176–9.
54 Interview with Emily Skillicorne, 16 June 2017.
55 Van Reyk, 'Life during wartime: nursing on the frontline at Ward 17 South at St Vincent's Hospital', *HIV Australia*, 12.1 (2014), 38–42 (at 39).
56 Fowler, *AIDS: don't die of prejudice*, p. 18.
57 See, for example, Clews, *Gay in the 80s*; Cook, 'Archives of feeling', p. 63.
58 See, for example, Julie Fish, 'Our health, our say: towards a feminist perspective of lesbian health psychology', *Feminism and Psychology*, 19.4 (2009), 437–53.
59 For a discussion of queer women's support of gay men during the HIV/AIDS crisis see 'His story, her story, it's all our stories', p. 37.
60 Interview with Farley Faragher, 7 April 2017.
61 Kevin M. De Cock and Nicola Low, 'HIV and AIDS, other sexually transmitted diseases, and tuberculosis in ethnic minorities in United Kingdom: is surveillance serving its purpose?', *British Medical Journal*, 314 (1997), 1747–51, tables 2 and 3.
62 Interview with George Jefferson, 14 August 2017.
63 For an account of this in the USA, see Carol Pogash, *As real as it gets: the life of a hospital at the center of the AIDS epidemic* (New York: Plume, 1992); Ronald Bayer and Gerald M. Oppenheimer, *AIDS doctors: voices from the epidemic: an oral history* (Oxford: Oxford University Press, 2002); Daniel J. Baxter, *The least of these my brethren: a doctor's story of hope and miracles in an inner-city AIDS ward* (New York: Mariner Books, 1998).
64 Virginia Berridge, 'AIDS and the rise of the patient? Activist organisation and HIV/AIDS in the UK in the 1980s and 1990s', *Medizin, Gesellschaft und Geschichte*, 21 (2002), 109–224.
65 Interview with Otto Best, 26 April 2017.
66 Reyk, 'Life during wartime'.

67 Interview with Elias Pound, 7 March 2017.
68 Interview with Aloysius Murphy, 4 February 2017.
69 Thomas S. Szasz, *The myth of mental illness: foundations of theory and personal conduct* (New York: Harper Perennial, 2010 [1961]); Ivan Illich, *Medical nemesis: the expropriation of health* (Marion Boyars Publishers, 1976).
70 Interview with Elizabeth Quayle, 4 August 2017.
71 Cave, 'Equipped to care', p. 55.
72 Interview with Marie Kelly, 22 February 2017.
73 Garfield, *The end of innocence*, p. 199.
74 David Miller and Len Curran, *The second sentence: the experience and needs of prisoners with HIV in HM Prison System, England and Wales* (London: HM Prison Service, 1991), p. 19.
75 Hughes, *Men and their work*; 'Work and the self'.
76 Prebble, 'Ordinary men and uncommon women', pp. 199–200.
77 Blake E. Ashforth and Glen E. Kreiner, ' "How can they do it?" Dirty work and the challenge of constricting a positive identity', *Academy of Management Review*, 24 (1999), 413–34.
78 Interview with Annie Crebbin, 2 October 2017.
79 Interview with Freda Rutter, 15 February 2017.
80 Interview with Elias Pound, 7 March 2017.
81 Goffman, *Stigma*.
82 Interview with Martha Munro, 17 February 2017.
83 This is discussed in the context of Ireland in Martin S. McNamara, Gerard M. Fealy, and Ruth Geraghty, 'Cultures of control: a historical analysis of the development of infection control nursing in Ireland', *Nursing History Review*, 21.1 (2013), 55–75 (at 65).
84 Interview with Bertha Brown, 6 May 2017.
85 Interview with Sarah Shimmon, 25 January 2017.
86 Interview with Freda Rutter, 15 February 2017.
87 Reyk, 'Life during wartime', p. 40.
88 Interview with Peter Pain, 20 March 2017.
89 Gideon Mendel, *The ward* (London: Trolley Books, 2017), p. 20.
90 Interview with Marsha Bausch, 13 March 2017.
91 Interview with Aloysius Murphy, 4 February 2017.
92 Interview with Peter Pain, 20 March 2017.
93 Elizabeth Lapovsky Kennedy, 'Telling tales: oral history and the construction of pre-Stonewall lesbian history', in *The oral history reader*, ed. by Robert Perks and Alistair Thomson, 2nd edn (New York and London: Routledge, 2006), p. 281.
94 Interview with Paaie Clague, 1 February 2017.
95 Interview with Margaret Kidd, 19 July 2017.

96 Catherine Dodds, 'HIV-related stigma in England: experiences of gay men and heterosexual African migrants living with HIV', *Journal of Community & Applied Social Psychology*, 16 (2006), 472–80.
97 On the AIDS epidemic in Edinburgh, see, for example, Stephen Mayes and Lyndall Stein, *Positive lives: responses to HIV – a photodocumentary* (London: Continuum International, 1993); interview with Elizabeth Quayle, 6 May 2017.
98 Interview with Hugo Pearl, 24 March 2017.
99 See, for example, Joe Wright, ' "Only your calamity": the beginnings of activism by and for people with AIDS', *American Journal of Public Health*, 103 (2013), 1789.
100 See, for example, Dickinson, *Curing queers*, pp. 179–99; Sally Hutchinson, 'Responsible subversion: a study of rule-bending among nurses', *Scholarly Inquiry for Nursing Practice: An International Journal*, 4 (1990), 3–17; Sally Hutchinson, 'Nurses and bending the rules', *Creative Nursing*, 4 (2004), 4–8.
101 Bobbi Campbell, 'Second National AIDS Forum', *San Francisco Sentinel*, 23 May 1983, p. 4. Robert 'Bobbi' Boyle Campbell, Jr. (28 January 1952–15 August 1984) was a public health nurse, the sixteenth person in San Francisco to be diagnosed with Kaposi's sarcoma (KS: a proxy for an AIDS diagnosis at the time), and the first to come out publicly as someone living with HIV/AIDS. He wrote regular articles in the *San Francisco Sentinel*, recounting his experiences and posting photos of his KS lesions to educate others. He also helped to write the first San Francisco safer-sex manual.
102 Quoted in Sage Sophier, *At home with themselves: same-sex couples in 1980s America* (Boston, MA: Spotted Books, 2014).
103 Interview with Luc Ferrier, 18 December 2017.
104 Cook, 'Archives of feeling', p. 67.
105 Interview with Hattie Price, 8 March 2017.

5

A phoney war? Health, education, and popular responses to HIV/AIDS in Wales, 1983–2003

Daryl Leeworthy

For one anxious caller to the Welsh AIDS Helpline in 1987, it was the probable impact of the widening health crisis on his cooked breakfast that prompted a tentative enquiry. Putting various bits of knowledge and gossip together, he wondered aloud whether the virus could be contracted from black pudding – which he liked to eat raw – since this was made from dried blood. As one public health worker in Wales later observed, 'this may appear amusing, but it illustrates the point that people draw their own conclusions when presented with information'.[1] Other enquiries and responses to surveys in the late 1980s and early 1990s noted widespread belief that the virus could be caught either from kissing or from coughing and sneezing, and a relative ignorance either of sexual transmission or infection from shared intravenous needles. This lack of understanding of how HIV/AIDS is transmitted continued into the twenty-first century, with a report in the Cardiff-based *South Wales Echo* published to mark World AIDS Day 2001 noting a stark increase in the number of positive test results in Wales that year. From around twenty a year for much of the 1990s, the figure increased more than three-fold in the first months of the new millennium.[2] Reflecting on the findings, one support worker noted that 'there are lots of myths out there and people in various social groups think it won't happen to them'.

But where did this attitude come from? And why, despite more than a decade of education programmes and public health initiatives in Wales, did it persist? The answers to these questions, and others which they prompt, lie in the experiences of those doctors and public health officials tasked with creating and leading the response to HIV/AIDS in the 1980s and 1990s, particularly in Cardiff and Swansea, and the challenges they faced. With relatively few reported cases in Wales and considerable pressure on health and local government budgets, not least instructions from central government to reduce staffing levels, the non-appearance of a crisis apparent elsewhere fostered a struggle between medical practitioners keen to prepare for what they regarded as the inevitable onset of urgent need, community campaigners keen to draw attention to those who had already been diagnosed and needed palliative care, and politicians and administrators.[3] In the words of Dr Donald Anderson, the leading consultant of public health in Cardiff at the time, the experience of HIV/AIDS in Wales at the end of the 1980s was 'reminiscent of the "phoney war" during the last months of 1939'.[4] In other words, despite the preparations made by medical personnel, there was still a belief that HIV/AIDS was, in some senses, an English disease, and that the virus would somehow avoid (or even ignore) the Welsh population.

Of course, it did not. Between 1984 and the summer of 1994, the Welsh Communicable Diseases Centre in Cardiff recorded 362 positive tests for HIV (see Table 5.1).[5] The clear majority – 197 cases – were men who had had sex with other men (MSM), with around eighty recorded among self-identified heterosexual patients. Blood transfusions represented the third-highest reason for infection (at almost sixty cases). Of the total figure, slightly more than one in three developed into instances of AIDS over the period.[6] Testing and subsequent HIV-positive identifications were overwhelmingly regionalised, with more cases in South Glamorgan (in effect, in Cardiff) than in any other county. In some parts of rural Wales, such as Pembrokeshire and Powys, there had been fewer than ten positive test results between 1984 and 1994. The Welsh results contrasted starkly with the situation in Scotland (even with the population difference taken into account), where more than 2,000 cases of HIV were recorded by the end of 1994, of which more than 600 had progressed on to AIDS.[7] Edinburgh, the Scottish capital, gained the unenviable moniker: the AIDS capital of Europe. This distinction between Welsh and Scottish experience continued throughout the 1990s and 2000s; by 2009, HIV diagnoses in Scotland were about double (as a percentage of the UK total) those in Wales.[8]

Table 5.1 HIV-positive results in Wales, 1984–94

Pre-1996 county	Post-1996 counties	HIV-positive results
Clwyd	Conwy, Denbighshire, Flintshire, Wrexham	37
Dyfed	Ceredigion, Carmarthenshire	15
Gwent	Blaenau Gwent, Torfaen, Newport, Monmouthshire	41
Gwynedd	Gwynedd, Ynys Môn	19
Mid Glamorgan	Merthyr Tydfil, Rhondda Cynon Taf, Caerphilly, Bridgend	16
Pembrokeshire	Pembrokeshire	<10
Powys	Powys	<10
South Glamorgan	Vale of Glamorgan, Cardiff	172
West Glamorgan	Swansea, Neath Port Talbot	55
Total		362

Adapted from: Olwen E. Williams, 'HIV ac AIDS – Y Sefyllfa Yng Nghymru/HIV and AIDS – the position in Wales', *Cennad: Cylchgrawn y Gymdeithas Feddygol/ Journal of the Medical Society*, 14 (1995), 68.

Unsurprisingly, the relative absence of HIV/AIDS cases in Wales together with their regionally disparate nature has been mirrored by historical disinterest, despite the revival of historical interest in HIV/AIDS elsewhere. Historians of Wales have yet to deal with the HIV/AIDS crisis or its consequences in a meaningful way, either through studies of epidemiology, social and political organisation, or through the potential of emotional history and the recovery of oral testimony.[9] This is despite a wealth of contemporary data collected by the Wellcome Trust-funded Project SIGMA led by sociologists Tony Coxon and Peter Davies, both initially based at University College Cardiff; epidemiological data collected by health boards and the government; and administrative material which forms part of the Welsh Office records at the National Archives.[10] As in earlier decades, of course, local archives remain difficult to access, closed off either through data protection legislation, cataloguing delays (themselves a symptom of austerity), or because relevant material has yet to be collected or deposited.[11] The present chapter represents an attempt to assemble a coherent narrative of Welsh responses to HIV/AIDS. Drawing on extant archival material, what follows suggests that, outside of Cardiff and Swansea, there was a strong degree of complacency concomitant with the idea of a 'phoney war'. In comparison with other political campaigns in Wales such as those addressing housing and unemployment (and with campaigns surrounding HIV/AIDS elsewhere), there was little cross-community engagement.

Three themes emerge in the present discussion: the work of the medical community and public health education, which was distinctive in its emphasis on young people and tempered by regional variation; the reactions of the general public and politicians, which were not always as hostile as Conservatives assumed; and finally the internal anxieties and reflections of gay men (and the extant sources *are* largely expressive of gay male voices) captured in telephone logs and interviews. These offer some indication of the personal response to the crisis in Wales. As an initial setting-out of the historical territory, the narrative below is undoubtedly tentative and subject to correction and clarification as further research is conducted. There is an inevitable stress on regional inequality and disparity, reflecting the absence of a unified Welsh approach to HIV/AIDS treatments and community support. In the words of one HIV/AIDS worker, spoken in 2007, 'local health boards across Wales aren't interested. I've rung each one of them to tell them what we do … and I was even met with giggles down the phone with one health board in mid-Wales. Only Swansea and Cardiff seem to get what we do.'[12]

Although this was hardly a uniquely Welsh challenge – urban facilities for the treatment of HIV/AIDS were generally better than rural provisions in any given context across the UK and elsewhere in this period – the regional imbalance was particularly pronounced in Wales. This was a time of increasingly nationalist politicking, with the idea of a single Wales promoted by politicians, commentators, the media, and the Welsh Assembly. That singularity was intended to challenge more traditional regional divisions and cultural affiliations, and to build up a Welsh polity based on all-Wales approaches.[13] Nevertheless, older divisions (north and south, urban and rural, richer and poorer) determined the extent of accessible healthcare and social services, and a person's likely experience of living with and seeking treatment for HIV/AIDS. Such imbalances between urban and rural provision, relative inequality, and take-up of services remained apparent into the twenty-first century even as all-Wales policy initiatives, such as the three-year PrEP trial launched in July 2017 and completed in June 2020, were undertaken. Careful consideration of the data, particularly as it relates to structural inequality and regional differences, will need to be undertaken in light of the now-routine availability of PrEP via the Welsh National Health Service.[14]

Medical manoeuvres

In 1993, researchers from Project SIGMA reflected on the tetchy relationship between gay men and sexual health services in Cardiff over the previous decade, noting that the local Genito-Urinary Medicine Clinic, based at the Cardiff Royal Infirmary, had an historically 'poor reputation'. It was unlikely to have been different elsewhere in Wales, although further research is needed to establish exact relationships and reputations.[15] This had a not-inconsiderable impact on the number of HIV tests administered, as well as treatment for other sexually transmitted infections in the city.[16] It invariably affected access to information, too. Alongside government campaigns and public health and sex education initiatives, there were articles in the local and national press which presented contradictory information about the virus and how to avoid transmission laced with hostility, moral finger-wagging, and fear, or a mixture of all three. Despite this, by the early 1990s support services in Cardiff (which was then administered as part of South Glamorgan) were well-developed with telephone helplines, a district coordinating centre, and a coordinating network which published a series of independent advice leaflets.[17] The further one lived from Cardiff, however, the less reliable and available information became, with student newspapers and community activism serving as the main source particularly in the north and west of Wales.

South Glamorgan Health Authority (SHGA) first discussed HIV/AIDS in the autumn of 1984 in response to growing public interest and the fact that the topic, in the words of the area's chief administrative medical officer (CAMO), was one of 'considerable national and local press interest at present'. In stating the authority's current position, the CAMO observed that 'the UK was on the verge of rapid increase in the numbers suffering with this disease, following trends in the USA'. Locally, two people had died of HIV/AIDS in the weeks leading up to the meeting – among the first such cases in South Glamorgan.[18] The authority's initial concerns focused on the potential transmission of infection through blood transfusions. This followed considerable behind-the-scenes discussion about the use of imported Factor VIII clotting agents from the USA and private recognition that a young haemophiliac being treated in Cardiff had likely been infected with HIV by that source.[19] The case was revealed in *The Mail on Sunday* on 1 May 1983 and discussed further in the *Daily Mail* and the *Daily Express* the following day.[20] A few months later, in an effort to quell public anxiety, Health Minister Kenneth Clarke asserted in the House of Commons that there was 'no evidence that AIDS is transmitted by blood products' and the head of the Cardiff Haemophilia Centre, Professor Arthur Bloom, told a meeting of specialists that, in his view, 'there was no need for patients to stop using the commercial concentrates [i.e., Factor VIII] because at present there was no proof that [they] were the cause of AIDS'.[21]

The introduction of heat-treated Factor VIII in 1984 provided a solution, alongside the first blood tests to enable diagnosis of HIV, but not before confidence in hospital procedures had been badly shaken.[22] A working group to deal with public concerns about blood donors and transmission of infection was thus established in South Glamorgan early in 1985, bringing together medical professionals, administrators, and councillors.[23] This marked a turning point in the seriousness with which HIV/AIDS was taken in the county, although attitudes were not always (in retrospect) enlightened; significant concern was expressed, for instance, that a proposed leaflet from the national Blood Transfusion Service did not include a specific question about whether a prospective donor was homosexual.[24] Members of the SGHA insisted that one be incorporated into the leaflet before it was released to the public.

Yet they also sought to provide funding for a testing laboratory at the University Hospital of Wales in Cardiff, despite a projected deficit of more than £4 million and a rate of underfunding from the Welsh Office of more than £2.5 million.[25] The authority also enabled half-a-dozen members of staff to be trained in the delivery of HIV/AIDS counselling and established a blood screening programme which had been used more than 20,000 times by the end of 1985.[26] A code of practice for health workers in South Glamorgan was issued the following year.[27]

Alongside efforts in South Glamorgan, a public health education programme was also established in West Glamorgan, focusing particularly on Swansea, and the Health Education Advisory Committee (HEAC) for Wales, which provided advice to the Welsh Office, established its AIDS sub-group in September 1985.[28] Membership of the latter included a deputy head teacher from a Gwent comprehensive school, the chief executive of the Welsh midwifery council, Tony Coxon from University College Cardiff, and health education officers from South and West Glamorgan (both of whom were coopted). The sub-group's recommendations to the Welsh Office, made in February 1986, included the creation of telephone advice and information lines, workshops for teachers and the media, the creation of publicity and education materials in English and Welsh, and a conference on counselling and confidentiality. By the time the report was accepted by the Welsh Office that summer, however, the UK government's own information campaign had begun, and Wales-specific elements were largely incorporated into or coordinated alongside national publicity. Nevertheless, in response to public opinion, a separate mechanism did come into existence – the Welsh AIDS Campaign – which was launched on 1 October 1986. Cardiff AIDS Helpline had been established a few months earlier.

As a counterpoint to the UK-wide 'Don't Die of Ignorance' tombstone advertisements, discussed further in Chapter 4, and particularly the fear that this campaign reflected and amplified, the Welsh AIDS Campaign set about trying to generate positive public information and awareness. Drawing on the expertise of the HEAC sub-group, a particular focus was schools and universities on the one hand and training medical personnel on the other. Perhaps the most notable achievement in the early months of the campaign was the production of one of the first bilingual AIDS information leaflets in Britain targeted at school children.[29] South Glamorgan Health Authority also produced videos such as 'Let's See What Tomorrow Brings'.[30] As Colin Griffiths, a member of West Glamorgan Health Authority's Health Education Unit and later director of the Welsh AIDS Campaign, observed in 1986, 'we hope this direct approach will temper the anxiety about AIDS which is obviously present but, hopefully, will be shown not to be justified'.[31] Towards the end of 1987, the Welsh Office changed its approach to AIDS and resolved that the Welsh AIDS Campaign would be merged with other public health initiatives into a single body – the Health Advisory Committee for Wales, later the Health Promotion Authority for Wales.[32] Consequently the Welsh AIDS Campaign 'sank without trace'.[33] Its final, high-profile intervention was a warning to rugby fans to 'stick to the beer and rugby, it's much safer than casual sex', which was issued ahead of the Scotland-versus-Wales Five Nations match at Murrayfield in Edinburgh in March 1987.[34]

Yet the Welsh AIDS Campaign's legacy was longer-lasting; its focus on education and awareness among young people can be seen across a number of initiatives in the early 1990s. One example is the work of the Welsh language youth movement, Urdd Gobaith Cymru (known informally as 'the Urdd'), which held its first national conference on HIV/AIDS in 1994.[35] Another is the work of sixth-form and further-education colleges to promote awareness and understanding in conjunction with World AIDS Day,[36] or, indeed, Health Promotion Wales' own World AIDS Day campaign from 1997, 'Young People: A Force for Change'.[37] Similarly, there were efforts by a small number of charities, businesses, and educational organisations to bridge the gap between public awareness and safety using board and card games and other forms of infotainment.[38] The Urdd launched its own Welsh-language AIDS information game in 1991.[39] These were the Welsh equivalents of a range of similar products created by local councils, health authorities, and charities elsewhere in Britain, such as 'Snakes and Ladders: A Game for Learning about AIDS/HIV', produced by the Hammersmith and Fulham Youth Service at the end of the 1980s, or 'Choices', produced by Lothian Regional Council's Community Education Service for use in Scotland.[40]

A phoney war? HIV/AIDS in Wales, 1983–2003   147

The creation of materials such as these was important, but impact on schools and in youth groups, together with availability, was relatively limited.[41] A survey of health-related teaching in Welsh primary schools conducted in 1993 noted that fewer than 40 per cent taught about HIV/AIDS; this compared with 50 per cent providing an 'education for parenthood' and three-quarters teaching about drug abuse. Sex education was delivered in three-quarters of infant schools and more than 90 per cent of junior schools, but the respective inclusion of material about HIV/AIDS was a mere 7 per cent and 45 per cent. Of those teaching pupils about HIV/AIDS, only a third believed it was 'adequately covered' in their school.[42] These figures had changed little by the time the next health promotion survey was conducted in primary schools in Wales in 1998; in fact, the number of schools that believed delivery of education about HIV/AIDS was adequate fell to below 30 per cent.[43] In secondary schools, by contrast, perhaps as a legacy of efforts to introduce educational resources in the 1980s, HIV/AIDS was regarded as being very important as a topic for health-related education. The adequacy of teaching was ranked considerably higher than in primary schools, with some 81 per cent of replies to a 1995 survey regarding it as such.[44] In retrospect, then, the initial wave of public awareness activity in the second half of the 1980s and the early part of the 1990s was unusual in its extent. The subsequent decline in support and organisational shuffling which took place in the second half of the 1990s and into the early 2000s ought not to be surprising, albeit just as community services were removed the number of people living with HIV/AIDS began to rise sharply (see Table 5.2).

Any survey of healthcare provision and education in Wales after 1997 must, inevitably, respond to the changes which took place because of devolution. The establishment of the Welsh Assembly, a devolved parliament for Wales, in 1999, following the referendum in 1997, transformed the way in which both health and education were managed, with greater stress on all-Wales approaches. Management of HIV/AIDS services was no different. In 2001, the Welsh Assembly Government launched its flagship HIV prevention programme in conjunction with the charity the Terrence Higgins Trust (THT) Cymru. The programme ran until 2009, informing the 2010 Sexual Health and Wellbeing Action Plan, the 2009 national

Table 5.2 HIV-positive individuals resident in Wales, 1997–2007

Year	Number	Year-on-year increase
1997	223	
1998	256	+33
1999	288	+32
2000	308	+20
2001	380	+80
2002	419	+39
2003	575	+166
2004	676	+101
2005	759	+83
2006	884	+125
2007	1,009	+125

Adapted from: Welsh Assembly Government, *Providing for the needs of people with HIV/AIDS in Wales* (Cardiff: Welsh Assembly Government, 2009), p. 2.

care pathway for HIV, as well as research carried out by AIDS Trust Cymru for the Stigma Index (now the Stigma Survey). The pathway provided, for the first time, a distinctive all-Wales programme of treatment and patient care, responding, of necessity, to the growing number of HIV-positive patients living in Wales – the figures exceeded 1,000 for the first time in 2007.[45] However, doubt must be cast on the success of these national programmes; access to services continued to be regionally inflected. Hospitals in Cardiff accounted for more than half of all attendances for HIV/AIDS treatment in 2003, and the figure still stood at 48 per cent in 2007.[46] Likewise of the eight hospitals across Wales able to provide specialist care, five were in the south and three in the north – none of the hospitals in Mid Wales offered these services.

That regional variations in both demand and provision of specialist services have continued to be a feature of the medical response to HIV/AIDS in Wales is noteworthy. Alongside these variations is the anxiety about healthcare provision revealed in the 2014 Stigma Survey. Although three in five of those questioned across Wales felt supported in primary care treatment, such as through their GP, some nonetheless 'feared being treated differently ... and some avoided care' entirely. This evasion was particularly true of dental care, with fewer than half of patients disclosing their HIV status to their dentist or dental practice.[47] This prompts the question of why, despite clear efforts on the part of policy-makers to implement national programmes, such concerns should continue to be expressed. Are they indicative of latent (and ongoing) hostility towards homosexuality and HIV/AIDS in Welsh society? Or, despite long-standing medical and educational efforts to the contrary, are they indicative of continued uncertainty (even ignorance) about the virus and methods of transmission? Perhaps, as Norena Shopland has suggested, the relative absence of discussion in Wales in recent years about HIV/AIDS has meant that individual anxieties and concerns have filled the vacuum left behind.[48] It is to these matters that we now turn.

Public hostility?

Of the many events associated with the HIV/AIDS crisis in Britain in the 1980s and 1990s, very few have drawn attention to Wales quite like the 1985 dispute at the Taliesin Theatre in Swansea involving the Gay Sweatshop theatre group and the theatre's own cleaning staff.[49] The cleaners had asked for additional rubber gloves, disinfectant, and protective clothing, ostensibly to ensure that they did not catch HIV/AIDS while cleaning toilets and other parts of the theatre; when this request was refused by the Taliesin's director the cleaning staff went on strike.[50] Although often presented as an example of homophobia (or, conversely, as was the case in contemporary tabloids, indicative of the threat posed by homosexuals), it turned out that the cleaners had been manipulated for the sake of publicity and the theatre's director faced considerable outrage from the student union at University College Swansea – including a motion of censure.[51] A more obvious, though less well-known, example of public hostility occurred ten years later in the North Wales community of Penmaenmawr, located between Conwy and Bangor. It was here that Tyddyn Bach, Wales' first HIV/AIDS respite centre, opened in 1997, but not without several years of debate and controversy after plans were first announced in 1995.[52]

As reported on television and radio, proposals for a respite centre in Penmaenmawr caused considerable consternation among some in the local population. 'The proposal', noted HTV News, 'has divided the seaside town … with objectors accused of being anti-Christian and bigoted'.[53] Petitions and planning objections were submitted by protestors, and local councillors vacillated between approval and rejection. 'Prejudice', remarked a member of the respite centre's organising committee, 'always has to bow to common sense'.[54] So it proved; in the spring of 1996, the centre was finally ratified by local councillors despite further protests, the resignation of two town councillors, and warnings that 'several local business people said they were selling up'.[55] Although the centre remained operational until 2012, it regularly faced financial difficulties and was rescued from closure in 2003 by a grant from the Welsh Assembly.[56] Nevertheless, as reported by the North Wales-based *Daily Post* in 2007, 'Wales's only HIV and AIDS respite centre has only been used by a Welsh sufferer twice since 2004 because it gets no statutory funding from either Westminster or Cardiff. Only English health authorities fund patients to visit Tyddyn Bach.' The centre manager, Philip Kearton-Smith, was recorded as saying that 'HIV charities shake their heads in disbelief when talking about Wales because our record on tackling the disease is so poor'.[57]

That failure reflected a relatively high degree of public ignorance, as well as some hostility, and a reduction in the extent of civic discussion about HIV/AIDS.[58] The first Welsh-medium television programme to mark World AIDS Day was not broadcast until 1997, for example, almost a decade after the inaugural World AIDS Day events in 1988.[59] Whereas the early 1990s had seen relatively widespread availability of advice and support services, with AIDS helplines established across Wales, the second half of the 1990s saw these steadily disappear together with the specialist knowledge provided. Indeed, the late 1990s and early 2000s were a period of not inconsiderable turbulence for HIV/AIDS services in Wales. This reflected, in part, changes in local government, health board administration, and the establishment of the Welsh Assembly's new structures. The decline in provision was most apparent in rural parts of Wales and in the postindustrial communities of the South Wales Valleys. The AIDS helpline for Powys was closed in 2002 after fourteen years, seemingly because the number of callers had plummeted – on some days, there were no calls at all. The closure of the Powys line mirrored the then-recent closures of the Gwent and Mid Glamorgan AIDS helplines, leaving only the North Wales and Cardiff helplines in place.[60] The Cardiff line merged with the Welsh branch of the THT in 2003.

Yet ignorance and confusion did not follow the retreat of community organisation, but had long been part of the Welsh experience to a greater or lesser extent.[61] Surveys conducted by Health Promotion Wales between 1987 and 1992 showed a range of misunderstandings about infection, responsibility, and consequences, with public attitudes and knowledge varying by gender, class, and sexuality.[62] For example, whereas almost a quarter of those aged over fifty-five who were surveyed in 1987 agreed that kissing a person with HIV could cause infection, only 10 per cent of those aged fifteen to thirty-four held the same view. Women were marginally more likely (17 per cent) to believe in the dangers of kissing compared with men (14 per cent), with a similar distinction between manual and non-manual workers (17 and 13 per cent, respectively). These figures had changed only slightly by 1992, with a fifth of those over fifty-five maintaining the view that kissing was dangerous. More positively, views on whether a person with HIV/AIDS should be able to live normally within a community improved significantly across the period. In 1988, just two-thirds of those surveyed agreed but by 1992 that had increased to 80 per cent. Women, non-manual workers, and those under thirty-five were more comfortable than those in other categories. Barely half of those over fifty-five agreed that HIV/AIDS patients should be able to live normally.

That attitude sat alongside growing hostility shown towards gay people in general among the Welsh population in the late 1980s and early 1990s. Tim Foskett, general secretary of the student's union at University College Cardiff and a leading figure in the Welsh campaign against Section 28, the Thatcher government's law against the promotion of 'pretended' (that is, LGBT) relationships, recalled in 1988 being taken aback by comments made to him during the 1987 Gay Pride march in Cardiff. 'There was fear in the faces of the onlookers ... and many moved away as we approached them with a leaflet. About forty people told us that we should be sent to the gas ovens.'[63] Survey results from 1988 showed that just under half agreed with the statement, 'I don't feel sorry for homosexuals infected with HIV because it is their own fault', with stark variations in class, gender, and generation. Men, older people, and manual workers were far more likely to agree than women, the young, and non-manual workers. There was a ten-point difference between the attitudes of young people (46 per cent agreed) compared with older people (56 per cent); by 1992 this had worsened, with 61 per cent of those over fifty-five agreeing that they did not feel sorry for 'homosexuals infected with HIV', compared with 47 per cent of those under thirty-five. Thus, whereas most of the Welsh believed that HIV/AIDS patients should be able to live normally, they still believed that infection among homosexuals was their own fault. It was a similar story for those infected through intravenous drug use.

Things have seemingly changed since the early 1990s. A study conducted by the polling company Ipsos Mori on behalf of the National AIDS Trust in 2014 noted that people in Wales 'tend to show a more supportive attitude towards HIV than people in other regions'.[64] Taking into account the relatively affluent cohort of respondents from Wales, which may be regarded (as Ipsos Mori itself suggested) as having a liberalising effect on the survey data, this observation was remarkable given the experiences and evidence discussed above. However, evidence from surveys conducted in the same period by Stonewall Cymru suggested that attitudes in Wales remained nuanced, even negative, with respondents observing that 'they can't talk openly to GPs and other healthcare workers and they are often too anxious that their confidentiality will not be protected'.[65] More than two-thirds noted that they had not spoken to their GP about HIV/AIDS, and two-thirds of this group insisted that they ignored the subject because they did not feel they had put themselves in risky situations.[66] As Stonewall Cymru concluded, 'these figures do raise grave concerns about the effectiveness with which hundreds of millions of pounds of public money have been spent on HIV awareness and prevention in recent years'.[67]

Risking it

One consistent theme evident in the survey data is that of risk, and inadequate social understandings of the virus. This evidence is, of course, by its very nature mediated and provides little indication of the personal emotions of queer trauma and how individuals negotiated the 'phoney war' which medical professionals perceived. How, for example, did an individual in Wales respond to the public information campaigns, the public hostility, and the social anxiety which followed the outbreak of the epidemic in the mid-1980s? Answers to these questions, or at the very least the evidential basis for the 'emotional guesswork' (to borrow Matt Cook's apposite phrase) involved, can be found in what Cook and Ann Cvetkovich have called 'archives of feeling' – those archival and ephemeral materials which shed light on emotions.[68] In his work Matt Cook has utilised the records of Mass Observation, which reflect personal submissions and responses to directives, whereas Cvetkovich drew upon a wide range of 'personal memories, which can be recorded in oral and video testimonies, memoirs, letters, and journals' since 'the memory of trauma is embedded not just in narrative but in material artifacts'.[69] Here I draw upon the extant logs of the FRIEND telephone helpline in Cardiff. Established in the early 1970s, FRIEND was a volunteer-run advice service which offered guidance on coming out, the practice of safer sex, and how to find and access queer venues across South Wales.[70] FRIEND also took forwarded calls from advice lines elsewhere including the Gwent AIDS Line, Icebreakers in Bristol, and Switchboard in London.[71]

The logs provide a range of (mediated) emotional 'data', as the following extract illustrates. It is the record of a call placed by a man who had recently returned to Cardiff after the death of his ex-partner's flatmate from AIDS. His ex-partner was also HIV-positive.

> Caller suffers from a stomach ulcer and in order to vomit had entered a public loo. He was then arrested for importuning by a plain clothes police officer. Discussed with caller the events leading up to the arrest and how he was treated by the police. He has been in contact with a solicitor in London who specialises in cases such as these and is going to see him [soon]. Caller broke down in tears several times during the call as he feels totally isolated and alone. Is concerned about his family finding out and also about his new work colleagues reading about it in the press. The call lasted approximately seventy minutes but he seemed a lot happier with things at the end.[72]

This extract conveys the psychology of this kind of telephone call, revealing, albeit succinctly, the processes of emotional outlay that are rarely captured by other sources. Much of the caller's own feeling, however, can only be guessed at since the log was compiled by the volunteer (there are no oral recordings).

FRIEND was often rung by young gay and bisexual men anxious about a sexual encounter, whether random or planned. Callers sought reassurance or guidance about potential infection, about safe sex (not least oral sex), and about the possibilities of enjoying more risqué sexual behaviour while limiting the risk of exposure to HIV.[73] A typical call in the early 1990s followed the pattern of revealing a sexual liaison after meeting another man at a bar, the anxiety which resulted from sex, discussion with their GP, and then placing the call to FRIEND to receive clarity from a queer voice. Volunteers took a cautious though not conservative line with callers, particularly as the crisis developed elsewhere, preferring to offer advice on safer sex and encouragement of low(er)-risk behaviour over the promotion of abstinence.[74] Concern about HIV/AIDS was occasionally framed by discomfort with aspects of the gay scene; callers discussed their disillusionment with demands placed on them regarding body image, promiscuity, and sexual behaviour.[75] One young man from Swansea initially called to lament the gay scene in the city before shifting to his forthcoming HIV test results. The latter, understandably, left him sounding 'flat and depressed'.[76]

Not every call was placed by an anxious individual concerned about the transmission of the virus to them. Parents and partners also rang to discuss their feelings: to express grief to a stranger, or to reflect on the breakdown of a familial relationship as the tensions involved in dealing with diagnosis and terminal decline proved too much.[77] In November 1993, to provide a typical example of the latter, Cardiff FRIEND received a call from a middle-aged woman from Bridgend, who had been referred by her local AIDS support service. During the discussion, it emerged that her son had been diagnosed with 'full-blown AIDS' and had left the house following a strong disagreement (the nature of which was not disclosed or recorded), providing no forwarding address or any means of further contact. The woman did not know whether her son was still alive, and unfortunately the log does not provide any clear indication as to the outcome of the search, either. Another such instance, from

April 1994, was a man ringing up seeking information about pubs and clubs in Cardiff that he could go to. He then revealed that his partner was in hospital dying of AIDS.[78] The emotional trauma of that passing away cannot be underestimated, nor should intentions be assumed – it may be that the caller needed time to deal with his own trauma. The telephone log, sadly, provides no indication of the volunteer's own response.

Given that the examples above reflect the situation in 1993 and 1994, a decade after the first diagnoses were revealed, to what extent were they different in form to earlier calls? Was there, for example, a steady hardening of attitudes among volunteers and callers as the epidemic developed? Evidence from the telephone logs suggests not. Instead, there continued to be a mixture of confusion, anxiety, trauma, and a need for advice. One call from 1987 was from a young bisexual man from Cardiff who had 'convinced himself he has AIDS'; he told the FRIEND volunteer that he was feeling guilty because of his infection and the effect it would have on his wife, whom he had not told about his bisexuality. As was common with this kind of call, the volunteer tried to offer reassurance and further advice about next steps. These included ringing the Cardiff AIDS helpline and arranging for a test at an STD clinic.[79] The hints, though not written down directly, that infection had come from casual encounters were by no means unusual. A significant number of the entries in the telephone logs in the 1980s as much as the 1990s refer to anxiety following cottaging or hook-ups at nightclubs and bars.

Calls from young men early in the coming-out process, or, indeed, at the beginning of it, provided opportunities to discuss HIV/AIDS prevention – an indication that FRIEND regarded itself, unofficially, as a necessary part of public health initiatives. One example is the following record of a call placed by a man from Abercynon in July 1987: 'Bisexual guy who wants to start exploring his gay sexuality. We talked about this for a while: his fears, interests, etc. I gave him the various places he could go to meet other gay people. We also had a brief chat about AIDS.'[80] Another such call, made the following year by a gay teenager from Anglesey who rang Cardiff to ensure no one on the island would find out about it, revealed the extent to which volunteers had to combat widespread naïveté about modes of infection, risk, and the dangers posed by the virus even when precautions were taken. It raised questions about the degree – and nature – of the sex education which he had received.

> Phoned us instead of any local number to find out if he could 'catch' AIDS from drinking cum out a Durex after the person he was with had screwed him. *Boy oh Boy!!* Well we discussed AIDS in general, AIDS in detail, and the health problems associated with such practices. He is only 17 and thought that as long as the guy was wearing a condom he couldn't catch anything rectally and couldn't catch anything orally anyway. We discussed all the issues he raised and he is better educated now than when he first called.[81]

Despite counsel to be cautious, it is clear that a variety of risks and values, from casual sex to promiscuity, were being adopted alongside what Peter Davies and Rayah Feldman have called 'minimization strategies [involving] rational, well-informed and sophisticated decisions about their behaviour'.[82] The risk to one's reputation when in the closet, for example, was measured differently to the medical risk involved in a casual encounter. Risks ranged from casual sex where safer sex was not being practised, to instances where different forms of safer sex were enjoyed – for instance, penetrative sex with a condom – to instances where those boundaries were blurred, such as oral sex without a condom.[83]

Conclusion

The twenty-year period between the first diagnosis in Wales in 1983 and the formation of THT Cymru in 2003 saw a remarkable transformation in the services made available for the treatment and public awareness of HIV/AIDS. Although Wales was by no means on the front line of the epidemic, circumstances nevertheless resulted in the provision of helplines, hospices, counselling services, educational information, conferences, and a respite centre. Despite the apparent 'phoney war', which resulted from the relatively slow growth in patient numbers in the 1980s and early 1990s, medical practitioners and health promotion educators in South Wales especially recognised the need to act to prevent widespread infection. Since 2001, however, the prevalence of HIV/AIDS has increased substantially, with three times the number of patients receiving treatment in 2010 in comparison with a decade earlier – a reflection, argues Public Health Wales, both of increased diagnosis and increased life expectancy.[84] Yet clinical reports of HIV in particular began to rise sharply in the early years of the new millennium – perhaps coincidental to the decline in community-based support services but, equally, perhaps not.[85] In fact, the sharpest rise in rates of infection in this period were between heterosexual men and women; in 2003, there were more than sixty reports of HIV transmission as a result of sex between men and women compared with around forty-five because of sex between men.[86] (This trend was first noted in 2002.)

There remains much more to be understood about the Welsh response to HIV/AIDS both in terms of community services, public responses, and the experiences of patients, physicians, educators, and policy-makers. Likewise, qualitative research into the personal experiences of queer men and women, using telephone logs of advice lines, oral histories, and Mass Observation, is an obvious area for growth in knowledge and understanding. In sketching a broad outline for wider research and discussion, I have sought to show that Wales deserves more attention from historians of HIV/AIDS because of the nuances involved in Welsh society, not least through regional variations, linguistic cultures, and shifting organisational approaches to healthcare and health promotion. But equally, HIV/AIDS deserves greater attention from historians of Wales and Welsh society because it allows for clearer scrutiny of the social democratic values to which, because of electoral politics, the Welsh are affiliated. In the end, there was no 'phoney war' against a 'gay plague' (or, indeed, an English disease) but rather a complex and changing series of responses to a developing situation. This, far more than hostility, ignorance, or absence, should serve as the framework for studying social and cultural reactions to HIV/AIDS in Wales.

Acknowledgements

For encouragement and guidance, I am grateful to Hannah J. Elizabeth, Janet Weston, George Severs, Patrick McDonagh, Tim Foskett, Jeffrey Weeks, and Matt Cook. Parts of this chapter were presented at a workshop at Birkbeck, University of London, and I would like to thank all the participants for their thoughts and responses. For archival support I am indebted to the Glamorgan Archives in Cardiff, the Richard Burton Archives at Swansea University, Special Collections and Archives (SCOLAR) at Cardiff University, and the Bishopsgate Institute in London.

Notes

1 Colin Griffiths, 'Welsh Pharmaceutical Conference: AIDS campaign must change direction', *Chemist & Druggist*, 17 October 1987, p. 787.
2 'AIDS cases treble in Wales', *South Wales Echo*, 1 December 2001, p. 7.
3 Glamorgan Archives, Cardiff (hereafter GA), D374/3, Bro Taf Health Authority Records, South Glamorgan Health Authority Minutes of Meetings, 19 June, 18 September 1985.
4 John Francis Skone, *The health services in South Glamorgan during 1986* (Cardiff: South Glamorgan Health Authority, 1987), p. 170.
5 Olwen E. Williams, 'HIV ac AIDS – Y Sefyllfa yng Nghymru/HIV and AIDS – the Position in Wales', *Cennad: Cylchgrawn y Gymdeithas Feddygol/Journal of the Medical Society*, 14 (1995), 68.
6 *Ibid.*, p. 69.
7 David Goldberg, Barbara Davis, Gwendolyn Muriel Allardice, Jim McMenamin, and Glenn Codere, 'Monitoring the spread of HIV and AIDS in Scotland, 1983–1994', *Scottish Medical Journal*, 41.5 (1996), 131–8. On HIV/AIDS in Edinburgh, see Chapter 6 in this collection.
8 Rachael Harker, 'HIV and AIDS statistics: UK', House of Commons Library, SN/SG/2210 (2012), p. 6. Available online at: https://researchbriefings.parliament.uk/ResearchBriefing/Summary/SN02210 (accessed 12 March 2019).
9 There are fleeting mentions in Martin Johnes, *Wales since 1939* (Manchester: Manchester University Press, 2012) and John Davies, *A history of Wales* (London: Penguin, 2007) but with little development. More problematically, Welsh experiences of HIV/AIDS are sidelined in Huw Osborne (ed.), *Queer Wales* (Cardiff: University of Wales Press, 2016). The most sustained treatment thus far is my own *A little gay history of Wales* (Cardiff: University of Wales Press, 2019). On the history of emotions, Thomas Dixon, ' "Emotion": the history of a keyword in crisis', *Emotion Review*, 4.4 (2012), 338–44; Matt Cook, 'Archives of feeling: the AIDS crisis in Britain 1987', *History Workshop Journal*, 83.1 (2017), 51–78.

10 Wellcome Library, GC260, 'Project SIGMA'; The National Archives, London (hereafter TNA), BD 133/15–16 and BD 133/38, 'Welsh Office, AIDS Steering Group'.
11 Virginia Berridge, 'Researching contemporary history: AIDS', *History Workshop*, 38 (1994), 228–34; Janet Weston and Virginia Berridge, 'AIDS inside and out: HIV/AIDS and penal policy in Ireland and England & Wales in the 1980s and 1990s', *Social History of Medicine*, 33.1 (2020), 247–67. See also Chapters 7 and 8 in this collection.
12 Mari Jones, 'Respite centre ignored', *Daily Post*, 25 October 2007. Available online at: www.dailypost.co.uk/news/local-news/respite-centre-ignored-2862327 (accessed 25 March 2019).
13 Dai Smith, *Wales: a question for history* (Bridgend: Seren Books, 1999); Johnes, *Wales Since 1939*.
14 Welsh government, 'Health Secretary Vaughan Gething announces all-Wales PrEP trial', 28 April 2017, available online at: https://gov.wales/health-secretary-vaughan-gething-announces-all-wales-prep-trial-0 (accessed 25 March 2019); 'Written statement: availability of Pre-Exposure Prophylaxis (PrEP) to prevent HIV', published 30 June 2020 at: https://gov.wales/written-statement-availability-pre-exposure-prophylaxis-prep-prevent-hiv (accessed 25 November 2021).
15 As an indication, see the information leaflet produced by Mid Glamorgan Health Authority in 1990 which presented HIV/AIDS support services overwhelmingly through the lens of intravenous drug use. Mid Glamorgan Health Authority, *Positive steps* (Bridgend: Mid Glamorgan Health Authority, 1990).
16 Peter M. Davies, Ford C. I. Hickson, Peter Weatherburn, and Andrew J. Hunt, *Sex, gay men and AIDS* (London: Falmer Press, 1993), p. 98.
17 South Glamorgan AIDS Network, *Positive care: a guide to care services for people affected by HIV/AIDS in South Glamorgan* (Cardiff: SGAN, 1993); South Glamorgan Health Authority, *An HIV/AIDS policy for South Glamorgan: facing the future together with confidence* (Cardiff: South Glamorgan Health Authority, 1992).
18 GA, D374/3: 21 November 1984.
19 'Letter regarding American Factor VIII sent to Department of Health and Social Services, 6 May 1983'. The evidence was made public in 2015 because of the Scottish Parliament's Penrose Inquiry and can be found online at: www.taintedblood.info/tb/tlfiles/DHSSLetterCardiffHaemophiliac6May1983.pdf (accessed 10 March 2019). The Penrose Inquiry material can be found at: www.penroseinquiry.org.uk (accessed 10 March 2019).
20 Susan Douglas, 'Hospitals using killer blood', *The Mail on Sunday*, 1 May 1983, p. 1; John Hamshire, 'Probe on imports of "killer

blood"', *Daily Mail*, 2 May 1983, p. 15; Douglas Orgill, 'The tragic disease shrouded in mystery', *Daily Express*, 2 May 1983, pp. 6–7.
21 Penrose Inquiry, Document PEN.015.0285. Available online at: www.penroseinquiry.org.uk/downloads/transcripts/PEN0150283. PDF (accessed 20 March 2019).
22 GA, D556/16: 19 December 1984.
23 *Ibid.*, 16 January 1985.
24 *Ibid.*, 20 February 1985.
25 *Ibid.*, 19 June, 18 September 1985.
26 *Ibid.*, 20 November 1985.
27 *Ibid.*, 15 January 1986.
28 What follows draws on Virginia Blakey, Richard Parish, and Debbi Reid, 'Health promotion responses to AIDS in Wales: the Welsh AIDS campaign', in *Responding to the AIDS challenge: a comparative study of local AIDS programmes in the United Kingdom*, ed. by Maryan Pye, Mukesh Kapila, Graham Buckley, and Deirdre Cunningham (London: Health Education Authority/Longman, 1993).
29 It was published in 1987. Welsh AIDS Campaign, *AIDS: what it means for young people* (Cardiff: Welsh AIDS Campaign, 1987). 'Youngsters get', *Liverpool Echo*, 26 February 1987, p. 19.
30 John Francis Skone, *The health services in South Glamorgan during 1987* (Cardiff: South Glamorgan Health Authority, 1988), pp. 177–8.
31 Colin Griffiths, Elizabeth Cruse, Joan Harries, Toni Williams, and Beverley N.C. Littlepage, 'AIDS – a health education approach in West Glamorgan', *Health Education Journal*, 44.4 (1985), pp. 172–3.
32 And finally, in its last guise, Health Promotion Wales.
33 Virginia Berridge, *AIDS in the UK: the making of policy, 1981–1994* (Oxford: Oxford University Press, 1996), p. 126.
34 'Rugby safer than sex', *Liverpool Echo*, 12 March 1987, p. 4.
35 National Library of Wales, Urdd Gobaith Cymru Records, 1997/C25, Gwyliau a Digwyddiadau/Holidays and Events, 1992–5.
36 HTV Wales News, 28 November 1990, 12 January 1992; HTV Wales, 'The Really Helpful Programme', 25 November 1993. The recordings are held at the National Library of Wales and were accessed there.
37 Health Promotion Wales, *World AIDS Day, 1st December: Young People: A Force for Change* (Cardiff, 1997).
38 HTV Wales News, 30 November 1988; as Hannah J. Elizabeth has shown, this was a very common form of flexible HIV/AIDS education. '[Re]inventing childhood in the age of AIDS: the representation of HIV positive identities to children and adolescents in Britain, 1983–1997' (unpublished PhD thesis, University of Manchester, 2016).

39 HTV Wales, 'Chwarter Call', 29 November 1991.
40 A copy of which is held at the National Library of Wales – item 94MC1767. A more extensive collection of HIV/AIDS teaching games, including 'Choices', is held at the Wellcome Library – my thanks to George Severs for pointing these out to me.
41 Anecdotally, sex education in my own primary and secondary school, both of which were in the South Wales Valleys, involved neither HIV/AIDS nor homosexuality.
42 Christopher Smith, Jane Frankland, Rebecca Playle, and Laurence Moore, 'A survey of health promotion in Welsh primary schools, 1993', *Health Education Journal*, 53 (1994), 241.
43 Suzanne McKeown, Chris Roberts, Chris Tudor-Smith, and Sue Bowker, 'Health promotion in Welsh primary schools, 1998', *International Journal of Health Promotion and Education*, 37.3 (1999), 83.
44 Chris Tudor-Smith, Chris Roberts, Nina Parry-Langdon and Sue Bowker, 'A Survey of Health Promotion in Welsh Secondary Schools, 1995', *Health Education* 97:6 (1997), p. 227.
45 Welsh Assembly Government, *Providing for the needs of people with HIV/AIDS in Wales* (Cardiff: Welsh Assembly Government, 2009).
46 *Ibid.*, p. 4.
47 Stigma Survey, *The people living with HIV: Wales* (London: Stigma Survey, 2015). This is available online at: www.stigmaindexuk.org/research-findings/ (accessed 25 March 2019).
48 Norena Shopland, 'Positively invisible women', *Oral History*, 35.2 (2007), 7.
49 The circumstances which occurred have been discussed many times and it is not my intention to provide comprehensive coverage here. For indicative discussions see Norena Shopland, *Forbidden lives* (Bridgend: Seren Books, 2017); Andy McSmith, *No such thing as society: a history of Britain in the 1980s* (London: Little, Brown, 2010); and on retrospective heritage sites covering Gay Sweatshop. Fullest coverage, drawing on university archives as well as contemporary press, is given in my own *A little gay history of Wales*.
50 *South Wales Evening Post*, 8 February 1985; *The Stage*, 7 March 1985, p. 23; NLW, HTV Wales Archive, 'Wales at Six: 19 February 1985'.
51 *Double Take*, 25 February 1985.
52 HTV News, 11 September 1995.
53 For reasons of space, I have not considered the religious and emotional dimensions invoked by this quotation.
54 HTV News, 13 December 1995.
55 HTV News, 15 May 1996.

56 'Wales's only HIV respite centre to shut down', *Daily Post*, 2 February 2012. Available online at: www.dailypost.co.uk/news/local-news/wales-only-hiv-respite-centre-2668621 (accessed 25 March 2019); 'Trust's crisis as HIV cases grow', BBC News, 1 December 2003. Available online at: http://news.bbc.co.uk/1/hi/wales/north_east/3253214.stm (accessed 25 March 2019).
57 Mari Jones, 'Respite centre ignored', *Daily Post*, 25 October 2007.
58 The hostility shown towards one North Walian patient led to him leaving for a new life in England. HTV, 'Face Value', 2 August 1990; S4C, 'Y Byd ar Bedwar/The World at Four', 4 June 1990.
59 S4C, 'Diwrnod AIDS y Byd/World AIDS Day', 1 December 1997.
60 'Rural area loses AIDS helpline after fall in callers', *Western Mail*, 4 September 2002, p. 9. The Cardiff helpline, the oldest in Wales, launched in July 1986; the North Wales helpline launched in 1989. HTV News, 13 January 1989.
61 Antony P. M. Coxon, *Between the sheets: sexual diaries of gay men's sex in the era of AIDS* (London: Cassell, 1996), p. 9.
62 The data discussed in the following section is drawn from Chris Roberts, Virginia Blakey, and Chris Smith, 'Changes in public knowledge and attitudes to HIV/AIDS in Wales, 1987 to 1992', *AIDS Care* 6.4 (1994), 413–21.
63 *Gair Rhydd*, 10 February 1988. Tim repeated this story to me when I interviewed him at the British Library in 2018 during research for *A little gay history of Wales*.
64 Ipsos Mori, *HIV: public knowledge and attitudes, 2014* (London: Ipsos Mori, 2014), p. 25.
65 Stonewall Cymru, *Gay and bisexual men's health survey Wales* (Cardiff: Stonewall Cymru, 2012), p. 3.
66 *Ibid.*, p. 14.
67 *Ibid.*, p. 15.
68 Ann Cvetkovich, *An archive of feelings: trauma, sexuality, and lesbian public cultures* (Durham, NC: Duke University Press, 2003); Cook, 'Archives of feeling'.
69 Cvetkovich, *Archive of feelings*, p. 7; some of the Mass Observation materials from the 1980s can be found online as part of the Observing the Eighties project: http://blogs.sussex.ac.uk/observingthe80s/ (accessed 25 March 2019).
70 The context of FRIEND and a fuller discussion of its creation can be found in my *A little gay history of Wales*; the telephone logs referred to below are held at the Glamorgan Archives in Cardiff.
71 GA, D320, Cardiff FRIEND, Telephone Log, 19 May 1987, for example.

72 *Ibid.*, 3 November 1993.
73 *Ibid.*, 16 April 1987.
74 *Ibid.*, 15 June 1993.
75 *Ibid.*, 5 March 1994.
76 *Ibid.*, 23 March 1993.
77 *Ibid.*, 29 September 1987.
78 *Ibid.*, 9 April 1994.
79 *Ibid.*, 4 April, 9 April 1987.
80 *Ibid.*, 21 July 1987.
81 *Ibid.*, 8 September 1988.
82 Peter Davies and Rayah Feldman, 'Selling sex in Cardiff and London', in *Men who sell sex: international perspectives on male prostitution and HIV/AIDS*, ed. by Peter Aggleton (Philadelphia, PA: Temple University Press, 1999), pp. 3–4.
83 Coxon, *Between the sheets*, p. 6.
84 Public Health Wales, *HIV and STI trends in Wales, surveillance report, April 2012* (Cardiff: Public Health Wales, 2012), p. 2. The precise figures were 383 cases in 2001 compared with 1,321 in 2010.
85 Public Health Wales, *HIV and STI trends in Wales, annual surveillance report, 2005* (Cardiff: Public Health Wales, 2005), p. 5.
86 *Ibid.*, pp. 5–6.

6

Recovering mothers' experiences of HIV/AIDS health activism in Edinburgh, 1983–2000

Hannah J. Elizabeth

> I am my own woman ... I have overcome a lot of obstacles. ... If you can't voice an opinion, make sure there is somebody who can do it for you or help you along the road.[1]
>
> Scottish HIV-positive mother, 1999

> When Clare feels sad about what HIV does to her mother, who is often tired and must have respite care for her illness, she eats jelly. 'I really like jelly,' she said. ... Clare is one of the forgotten victims of a disease that came to Edinburgh in the early 1980s when the city was flooded with cheap heroin.[2]
>
> Aileen Ballantyne, *Sunday Times* journalist, 1998

This chapter traces how healthcare workers and HIV-affected mothers responded to the AIDS crisis in Edinburgh in the last two decades of the twentieth century. In particular, it examines how women's health needs and needs as carers were met by the creation of new organisations and resources. It explores the ways the lives of HIV-positive mothers in Edinburgh were shaped by interdisciplinary collaborative HIV/AIDS care and activism born out of the daily fight for resources, information, space, and empathetic treatment for women and their families. Activism such as this was often indistinguishable from survival or best practice, occurring in the clinic and the home, in acts of care performed by medical practitioners and family members, and through the voicing and documenting of needs. This work can be traced through a wide variety of texts and archives, and was at the very least a backdrop for many women's experience of HIV and AIDS in Edinburgh.

To focus the analysis, I examine the creation of the Paediatric AIDS Resource Centre (PARC) in Edinburgh, alongside some of the items the centre published and disseminated, as well as other forms of activism the centre supported. PARC's activities were varied, from creating factual leaflets to facilitating training and publishing picture books, shaping mothers' experiences of HIV/AIDS activism both subtly – by training volunteers and broadening general HIV knowledge among the caring professions – and more directly by providing resources to them and their children. It is this textual history, alongside the words of HIV-affected mothers and the professionals who worked with them, that this chapter adds to the history of HIV/AIDS which has too often missed these stories. Following the example of those working with HIV-affected families at the time, I also pay particular attention to how the emotional needs of those affected by HIV were met, attending to the importance of familial bonds between mothers and children. I begin by sketching the landscape of care available to HIV-affected mothers in Edinburgh before PARC was founded, outlining the tone of media coverage, the medical and social care facilities which emerged, and the gap PARC was created to fill.

The chapter ends by examining some of the texts PARC created to facilitate conversations between HIV-affected parents and children after 'it dawned on social workers that [they] ... might actually have a lot more children affected by HIV rather than infected by HIV'.[3] I demonstrate how PARC, in responding to a much-expressed need for resources, addressed the perpetual parenting question: what do we tell the children? Analysing PARC alongside the testimony of HIV-affected mothers and those that worked with them allows us to begin the work of recovering mother's experiences of HIV/AIDS, redressing a gap which has too long existed in the historiography.

The sources on which this chapter draws are diverse. For a variety of reasons, some of which are discussed below, the experiences of HIV-affected mothers living in Edinburgh in the 1980s and 1990s form an especially scattered archive. Their voices can be found in contemporary mainstream press, AIDS care newsletters, social work training manuals, medical journals, oral histories, picture books, and anthologies of their testimonies, to name but a few. As the contrasting quotations at the start of this chapter show, some texts present assertive statements from HIV-affected mothers and children, speaking to the networks of care that empowered them. In other contexts, their words appear only as bleak illustrations of profound tragedy, presented in service of an agenda which gave little space to their agency.

While each text offers a valuable glimpse of the lived experiences of HIV-affected motherhood, they all present their own difficulties in terms of their mediated nature and the power dynamics which coloured the disclosures they deliver. In some cases, mothers are spoken about rather than speak, their experiences described in aggregate or fictionalised. Other texts offer examples of the way disclosure of one's HIV status could be empowering, allowing access to much-needed resources or even acting as a form of activism itself. Indeed, disclosure of one's HIV status and the experiences which attended it were so important that some texts devoted pages, chapters, or entire volumes to this form of testimony. In many of the texts that I draw on below, however, the agency and motivations of the speaker are harder to discern. Social work manuals and childcare training texts contain letters, poems, and drawings which allowed HIV-affected and HIV-positive mothers and children to speak back to the health and social care community who worked to meet their needs. At the same time, the textual placement and case study presentation style used in such texts had the potential to turn such salvos into means rather than ends – experiences to learn from rather than sit with. As a historian I am unsure of, and uncomfortable with, the production context of such traces, and yet I want to give them space in the histories I tell, to return them to circulation rather than leaving them languishing unread in social work manuals that no one is using anymore. This is part of the recovery to which the title of this chapter speaks.

As thinking in HIV-related social work developed, workers began to use the term HIV-affected to refer to those 'infected or those who live in a family or community where ... carers, relatives or peers have the virus, which will have emotional, social or economic consequences'.[4] As I have argued elsewhere, I use this term in part for its breadth and ambiguity, echoing the instructional social work texts which form part of my archive.[5] HIV-affected encompasses both service users and service providers, and, in the case of texts, producers and their audiences, acknowledging the complex production context of the texts under analysis. The ambiguous relationship between the producers of these texts and their audience is in part the product of the liminal space that health and social care workers who worked with HIV-affected people came to occupy in this period. The HIV/AIDS worker quickly became 'HIV-affected', experiencing 'courtesy stigma' as fears of casual transmission persisted, and they became emotionally compromised by the difficulties associated with their work.[6]

In focusing on mothers' experiences, there are stories which can and cannot be told. Children's needs do feature, but the voices of other key individuals in the lives of HIV-affected mothers have not found space here. Partners, parents, extended family, friends, and lovers all shaped the experiences of HIV-affected mothers, as did the myriad health and social care workers who engaged HIV-affected families. While this chapter acknowledges the ways that queer expertise in fighting for the rights and needs of HIV-affected people profoundly shaped the delivery of HIV care and education in Edinburgh, the voices of LGBTQ activists require more space than this chapter allows. These are histories we still need to write, and I offer this chapter as a starting point in larger project which will write the interconnected history of HIV-affected family life in Edinburgh.[7]

Early responses in the 'AIDS capital of Europe'

At the time of writing, most published histories of HIV/AIDS in the United Kingdom (UK) are largely inattentive to regional specificity, and England often stands in for all four nations.[8] Moreover, owing to the historiography's focus on media representations, policy-making, and gay men's activism, such work is particularly representative of events and experiences in the south of England and London especially, rather than offering a fuller national history of the impact of the virus.[9] Regional specificities are myriad, and in ignoring them we neglect the histories of those who fought on the local as well as the national scale to combat the spread of the virus and its social and its morbid effects. These differences occurred on the grand scale in terms of policy-making and tax spending, but are starker still when we consider differences along a more modest scale: the who, what, when, where, and how of service provision for HIV-affected people. As has been well documented, the 'Don't Aid AIDS' campaign filled television screens across the UK with tombstones, and doormats with 'Don't Die of Ignorance' pamphlets, in 1987. These striking gestures from a national government in search of a cost-effective solution to HIV/AIDS were by no means the most successful or most important assault on the problem in the UK. Indeed, in many ways these grand efforts were woefully deficient in the face of a new illness. Such attempts to halt the spread of HIV through mass education were lacking in details and left the needs of those already infected or affected by the virus largely unmet.

Scotland's experience of HIV/AIDS, while regionally and internationally inflected and influential, was demographically, culturally, and politically distinctive. For example, of those with HIV in Scotland by 1991, 63 per cent had contracted the virus through either heterosexual intercourse or needle sharing, versus 24 per cent for the UK as a whole.[10] Edinburgh, as a city, was disproportionately affected by the HIV/AIDS crisis in the early 1980–1990s, earning it the unhappy title of 'AIDS capital of Europe'.[11] Edinburgh's crisis followed a different pattern from that which was unfolding in London, with new infections predominantly occurring among intravenous (IV) drug users and heterosexuals.[12] While statistics from this period are problematic – recording sex and gender as a binary, sexuality as essentially heterosexual or *other*, and rarely recording ethnicity or age – there are some aspects of Edinburgh's HIV epidemiology we can glean. The retrospective testing of blood samples in 1985 (collected from IV drug users before the growing epidemic was recognised) indicated that between 1,000 and 1,500 IV drug users seroconverted in the city of Edinburgh between the summers of 1983 and 1984.[13] By 1985, 50 per cent of 'known' injecting drug users, meaning those engaged by social, medical, or criminal justice workers, were HIV-positive.[14] By 1987 Edinburgh accounted for 30 per cent of all cases of recorded HIV among women in the UK, and Edinburgh had the highest rate of recorded HIV cases in the UK overall.[15] By 1993, there were 500 'known' HIV-affected children with complex care needs in Edinburgh.[16]

Social workers working with HIV-affected people in the 1980s and 1990s stressed that all estimates were likely to be missing many HIV-affected families. What's more, the vagaries of the epidemiological statistics available failed to record a variety of forms of intersecting need, caused by some of the demographic specificities which shaped the experiences and health outcomes of HIV-affected people. Indeed, in 1991, social worker and expert on the familial dimensions of HIV/AIDS Naomi Honigsbaum charged the unclear collecting and reporting of statistics with creating a 'falsely optimistic view that infectivity in children is statistically insignificant'.[17] Children affected by – rather than infected *with* – HIV were even less likely to receive statistical acknowledgment. Parental status was not always asked of newly identified HIV-positive adults, and children with a non-parental close relationship to someone living with HIV or AIDS largely went unrecorded, with some children even going uncounted when it was the father, rather than the mother, who had the virus. These statistical deficiencies affected the distribution of funding for HIV-affected families, essentially hiding the social needs of those HIV-affected family members who did not fall under the purview of medical treatment or transmission prevention. Despite these quantitative difficulties, it is clear that in Edinburgh women and children were affected by, and in some cases infected with, HIV in higher numbers than elsewhere in the UK. As a result, Edinburgh became a hub of activism and expertise as the HIV-affected and those who cared for them scrambled to address previously unmet needs.

National education campaigns produced by the Health Education Council, Department of Health and Social Security (DHSS), and, later, the Health Education Authority across the late 1980s and early 1990s discouraged unprotected sex and IV drug use. However, the needs of those at risk because they were surviving through sex work, or already dependent on IV drugs, or those already positive or caring for someone positive also needed to be addressed. From 1985 to 1986 England's Central Office of Information ran the 'Heroin Screws You Up' campaign, deploying 'shock horror' tactics. This was matched in Scotland by the more optimistic Scottish Health Education Group campaign 'Choose Life, Not Drugs'.[18] Both were aimed at reducing IV drug use, but met criticism for failing to grasp the social deprivation which led many to become drug users, or the circumstances which resulted in persistent dependence.[19] Similarly, when the DHSS attempted to tackle AIDS with its foreboding 'Don't Aid AIDS' campaign, running from 1986 to 1988 and featuring the 'Don't Die of Ignorance' television advert balefully voiced by John Hurt, Lothian Health Board (LHB) offered Edinburgh's citizens their own health campaigns. LHB and the Lothian Regional Council HIV/AIDS team first ran the inclusive 'AIDS Concerns Us All' campaign, commenced on World AIDS Day 1988, then a few months later launched the similarly upbeat 'Take Care' campaign, begun with much fanfare on Valentine's Day 1989.[20]

While large-scale national and local government public health campaigns attempted to prevent new infections through a variety of media – from TV and radio to posters on buses – the high rates of HIV among women in Edinburgh meant the city rapidly became host to numerous charities and organisations focused on women and their families already affected by the virus. These organisations aimed to prevent new infections, but also strove to meet the emotional, medical, housing, care, and educational needs of those already living with the virus. It is the meeting of these needs that I examine below, foregrounding the specificity of women's experiences of HIV/AIDS in Edinburgh when the city's crisis was at its zenith.

Media-mediated motherhood

'This child has inherited Britain's most terrifying disease – from its mother', declared the tagline of a 1986 *Daily Mail* article titled 'My guilt when they said I'd given my baby AIDS'.[21] I begin by examining this lengthy article, which was featured in the paper's women's supplement *FeMail*, because it offers a typical example of the stigmatising representation of Edinburgh's AIDS crisis and HIV-affected motherhood in the 1980s.[22] Historians must pay attention to articles like this precisely because they are exactly the kind of problematic documents from which researchers might seek to recover mothers' voices. They offer, albeit in a highly mediated fashion, glimpses of some of the factors which shaped the experiences of women living with HIV in Edinburgh in this period, revealing the context which made the creation of PARC so necessary. Moreover, this kind of stigmatising representation formed the context for many of the empowering educational interventions made by HIV-affected mothers and those that loved and cared for them. It offers a flavour of how the reading public might have encountered Edinburgh's AIDS crisis and the mothers it affected. I critique it here to demonstrate the agency-stripping pessimism against which women fought, and to offer a little of the texture of the world built by a press intent on sensationalising AIDS to the detriment of those affected by it.

As I have argued elsewhere, following Steven Kruger, disease narratives and particularly those relating to pandemics allow 'an ordering of events', constructing a sense of 'meaning' or 'reality' which appears to have an authored coherence, 'as though its cause and ultimate reason ... might be uncovered'.[23] This 'intentionality' in turn allows for 'moralized understandings', confining culpability and innocence to certain behaviours and characters.[24] Representations of AIDS, Kruger argues, can be divided into two interrelated major narratives: the macrocosmic and the microcosmic. The former is concerned with an 'epidemiological or population narrative', often following the 'historical trajectory of the epidemic' in search of an 'origin', then tracking the epidemic's 'progress', the 'spread of the disease', and finally the 'explosion of cases' within a particular population – an 'at-risk' group – which will finally, in the 'worst-case scenario', result in an 'apocalyptic spread of disease' wherein the virus breaches the boundaries of the 'risk groups', entering the 'general population'.[25] In the latter narrative, an individual's relation to the illness is represented, charting from the point at which contact with the virus is made to the positive test result, the development of symptoms, the AIDS diagnosis, and finally death. Within this microcosmic narrative of AIDS, '[p]assivity is imputed at all stages ... except the initial stage, where, too often, a certain "culpable" activity is associated with the exposure to HIV'.[26] It is this latter narrative which the *Daily Mail* article follows.

The article states that 'innocent baby ... little Jamie ... is one of 29 babies to be infected in the womb because of a parent's drug abuse', firmly placing responsibility on his 'frail' mother and her 'drug addict husband'.[27] Jamie's mother Lorraine is then quoted in confirmation of this guilt: 'Every morning I wake up and blame myself ... It makes me angry that Jamie has been the innocent victim of our drug abuse'.[28] Personal culpability for the spread of HIV thus established, the article moves from the intimate blame narrative between Lorraine, her husband, and their baby Jamie to take in the wider epidemic: 'Lorraine is just one of a growing number of Scottish heroin users who have made Edinburgh Britain's drug and AIDS capital.'[29] Edinburgh was first described as Europe's AIDS capital in 1986, in part because the epidemiological significance of its drug-using population was identified relatively early on in its AIDS epidemic, leading to vocal health workers and drug users calling for efforts to mitigate the crisis.[30]

In the *Daily Mail* article, we are told that:

> It is in Edinburgh that the most tragic maternity clinic in the county is to be found. Ward 7A at the Edinburgh City Hospital appears at first sight to be like any other post natal clinic, with the sound of babies' laughter filling the room, but over all lies a pervading sense of terror and guilt.[31]

Among those on the ward is Sylvia, twenty-three, who 'is plagued by infinite guilt for what she has done to her innocent child'.[32] Quoted in *FeMail*, she explained that 'Jonathan's birth was weird. All the doctors had goggles over their heads like space helmets. I supposed they were to protect them from my disease. It was the first time I had met people who were so terrified of AIDS.'[33] Sylvia then goes on to explain the conditions of her care, offering a familiar tale of the isolating experience of contact-free care in an atmosphere of fear: 'In hospital I felt like an outcast, eating off plastic plates and drinking out of plastic cups. I felt like a leper. I couldn't wait to leave hospital.'[34] At no point does the article furnish readers with the knowledge that HIV could not be casually transmitted by social contact, despite this having been established as early as 1983.[35]

The article allows Sylvia the opportunity to explain something of what it was to be an HIV-affected mother, although this is filtered through a veil of blame and hopelessness. 'I'm dreading the day he goes to school', Sylvia is quoted as saying,

> … and the day I have to tell him he has AIDS. How do you tell a wee boy that he has only a 50% chance of life? And how do you tell him that it is all the fault of Mum and Dad? I don't even know, I might not have to. In five years' time we might both be dead.[36]

Worries about how to disclose to children that they or their parents were living with HIV or AIDS were so common an experience that by the 1990s a variety of texts had been created to help HIV-affected parents make such disclosures, many published by PARC. For Sylvia, as one of the first identified HIV-positive mothers, such resources did not yet exist. The article offers a hint of hope for the future when it turns to the discussion of HIV/AIDS experts Drs Mok and Brettle and their work in the City Hospital's 'AIDS clinic'. They quote Mok's explanation that the

> general medical attitude to these mothers is full of gloom and despondency. They believe they have nothing to look forward to but death. For the first time we are offering them something positive. We tell them their future is in their hands.[37]

But this empowering message was merely employed by the *FeMail* article to create a sense of contrasting drama as rising hopes are dashed. It asks in response to Mok's hope, 'But for all their hard work, is their clinic really a success?', before ending with Sylvia's despairing words, 'when you think about it, there's not much they can really do. I will never stop feeling terrified and guilty. And whatever they say, I know it's more likely that I will die than live. What can you say to that?'[38] The gloomy end of the article belies its voyeuristic intent, eliciting sympathy in its general readers while painting AIDS as an isolating and devastating illness happening elsewhere. Although the *Daily Mail* showed little care for the disheartening effects of this kind of narrative, those involved with Edinburgh's paediatric AIDS clinic were working hard to bring an end to the isolation and fear the article described.

Taken on its own, the City Hospital's Paediatric AIDS clinic might not have felt like a success in the face of an illness which appeared to be overwhelming both individual patients and carers, as well as the health and social service sector more broadly. But the clinic was not on its own. Rather, it formed part of a network of emerging services intended to meet the health needs of HIV-affected mothers. These networks, and the actors like Mok who played pivotal roles within them, became the genesis for organisations such as small charities, support groups, campaign networks, or research groups. Indeed, the expertise which accumulated around the health practitioners and mothers at the City Hospital's AIDS clinic would eventually form the basis of PARC, an organisation working to create and disseminate empowering knowledge for HIV-affected mothers and those that worked with them.[39]

'We had a mission': Edinburgh's emerging expertise around HIV-affected motherhood

From October 1985, consultant paediatrician Dr Jacqueline Mok had responsibility for monitoring and following up all babies born to HIV-positive women in the Lothian. During an oral history collected in 2018, Mok recalled that when she was asked to 'look after these children born to mothers with HIV' in the first HIV clinic dedicated to the care of children in the UK, she responded by questioning, 'what do I know about that?' Public health consultant Dr Helen Zealley, who had requested Mok take up the role, replied by pointing out that nobody else knew anything either.[40]

While HIV in children was recognised in 1982, knowledge on paediatric HIV, rather than AIDS, remained scarce in 1985.[41] Some doctors were still too scared to work with HIV-positive expectant mothers because, as Zealley explained, 'there's a lot of blood around when people deliver, people were terrified of blood'.[42] Mok herself joked that the request to set up an HIV clinic for mothers and babies was also to 'risk your life and be infected', and recollects being told by other doctors to 'just keep your clinic down at the city hospital, we can't have them at Sick Kids', Edinburgh's dedicated children's hospital.[43] Despite this atmosphere of fear, uncertainty, and what Mok described as 'gloom and doom', over the next few years Mok was among a small number of health workers in the Lothian tasked with figuring out how to meet the needs of HIV-affected families.[44] Eventually Mok became both an expert in the care of HIV-affected mothers and children, and their educational needs, and in her role as co-director of PARC ensured that HIV-affected, as well as HIV-positive, mothers and children had access to the emotional and educational resources they wanted.

Trying to bridge the knowledge gap around HIV-positive mothers and babies, Mok travelled to New York, New Jersey, and Florida in 1985 to look at what had been set up for children there. However, she found that while expertise was developing globally, little was known about HIV-positive mothers and babies, rather than mothers and babies living with AIDS. Many mothers in Edinburgh were found to be HIV-positive but not yet ill, so the new services were focused on monitoring healthy mothers and babies, as well as treating AIDS. It is worth noting that those mothers who discovered their serostatus during pregnancy were generally advised, where medically and legally permissible, to terminate their pregnancy, in line with advice issued by the Royal College of Obstetricians and Gynaecologists in 1986.[45] Indeed, as one Scottish HIV-positive mother diagnosed at three months pregnant later recalled,

> the medical staff at the time, were very negative. They made me feel worthless really. ... Everyone expected me to get an abortion, medical staff, the whole lot. ... the way I was treated at the time made me feel worthless.[46]

Mothers were advised to terminate their pregnancies in part because it was believed, in the early years of the AIDS crisis, that pregnancy would accelerate the speed at which HIV-positive women developed AIDS, and that mother-to-baby transmission was around 50 to 80 per cent with the prognosis for paediatric AIDS very poor.[47] Despite this advice, many HIV-positive mothers continued their pregnancies and HIV-positive women continued to become pregnant, so the need for dedicated services in Edinburgh grew as the 1980s progressed.

Many HIV-positive mothers' experiences of birth were negatively affected by stigma, barrier nursing procedures, the uncertainty of mother-to-baby transmission rates, and the resultant pressure to terminate pregnancies. Frequently, HIV-positive mothers reflected on the continued feelings of guilt instilled in them by the media and the medical profession. Many also spoke of the anger they felt after experiencing poor treatment during birth. One mother who recalled a particularly traumatic birth described it, and the aftercare she received, as 'the worst four days I have ever experienced', and acknowledged a lasting sense of culpability after the birth: 'I felt really guilty. In my head I saw it as some form of abuse, because I didn't realise at the time that she [her baby] might lose the positive antibodies.'[48] Owing to these experiences, and other vulnerabilities common to HIV-positive mothers in Edinburgh, those working with HIV-affected families had to tread carefully and rebuild trust where it had been damaged. While ties between the voluntary, activist, and statutory sectors were key to achieving this, adaptation and research into what mothers actually wanted from health and social care services were also fundamental.

Postnatal and paediatric care took place inside and outside the hospital clinic, with home visits forming a key aspect of the care and monitoring which structured the first few months of HIV-positive mothers' and babies' lives after a new birth. At first Mok and Dr Ray Brettle (infectious disease consultant at the City Hospital with an interest in IV drug users' health) thought they should hold 'a family clinic' so that 'when the parents would come they would bring their children. But because the parents didn't come … the sort of family clinic became a mish mash of some clinic appointments and mainly home visits.'[49] Established in 1986, initially the paediatric counselling and screening clinic ran 'two sessions a week', but Mok explained that these 'became community based because sitting in my clinic at the City Hospital and expecting these very chaotic families to bring their children just didn't work'.[50] Indeed, less than 20 per cent of families used the Paediatric HIV Service outpatient clinic at Edinburgh City Hospital, with many preferring the home as both more 'convenient' and 'less distressing'.[51] Other families decided to keep the home 'a sanctuary of normality for the child, free from painful interventions', choosing instead to use a general practitioner (GP), health visitor clinic, or their child's nursery.[52] By allowing parents to choose the location of clinical encounters, as far as possible, much-needed trust could be built and the burden of surveillance lessened.

While locations differed, regimes of medical testing, surveillance, and treatment were fairly similar. When the European Collaborative Study (ECS) into paediatric HIV was initiated in 1985, Edinburgh was one of the first centres to join, quickly enrolling babies into the cohort study.[53] The standard testing protocol for babies included in the ECS was onerous. Each baby, as Mok explained,

> needed something like a follow-up at one week, three weeks, six weeks, and then six-weekly until six months, three-monthly until aged two years, and then six- to twelve-monthly. We also had to speak to the mothers in the antenatal period to seek their consent, to explain to them about the purpose of the study. Nobody actually withdrew consent. They were all very willing. They were very interested. Actually they were very thankful that somebody was interested in them and their children.[54]

As the numbers included in the cohort study grew, funding was sought from the Scottish Office to pay half of Mok's salary and to pay for a research fellow. The biweekly nurse-run hospital clinic sessions were replaced with a full-time health visitor to help facilitate home visits, or, as Mok put it with a little exasperation, 'we actually did home visits to actually make sure that we could actually see these children'.[55] From Mok's perspective, home visits were a laborious way of meeting the needs of difficult patients, who were challenging to work with even with this added intervention.

> Unfortunately there was some who would continue to use [drugs], and those were the ones that you never knew when you went to see them, if, you know, they would be awake, what state they would be in, whether they would be cooperative. [56]

Mok's perspective is that of a medical practitioner stepping outside the clinic to meet the needs of her patients and their families. However, her testimony acknowledges some of the reasons why HIV-affected families might have resisted interventions. The predominant route of infection for HIV-positive adults in contact with the family clinic was needle sharing, and so many of the families involved in the study had a history of poor relations with statutory services, which was often compounded by a difficult birth experience.[57] Moreover, the fear of children being taken into care often became a reality for those parents who were unable to recover from their addiction, prompting additional anxieties about dealing with authority figures such as health visitors. Other HIV-positive mothers found interventions frustratingly limited and the uncertainty around treatment exhausting. Writing in 1989 from Edinburgh's Brenda House rehabilitation centre, one HIV-positive mother offered the following angry poetic response to well-meaning medical advice, later included in a social work manual.

> ... Tell me now will I die
> Well we have this brand new drug to try
> Would you like it now?
> Would you like it later?
> When you're being sick an' shittin' through a grater
> ... Eat well, eat good they say
> On fuckin' what, 10p a day?[58]

As well as the intrusion of health workers and sometimes social workers into the home, the physical nature of tests also caused difficulties. Mok admitted that 'it was a lot of blood' being taken from small babies. While mothers were often 'very compliant … it was the fathers that we got the most flack from. … they either just left during the blood-letting, "oh I canea take this", you know, these great big men, or they would get really angry'.[59] Mok remembers being shouted at when attempts to take blood from babies failed. The pressure to get it right increased by the presence of distressed parents.

Despite these difficulties, by entering the home and offering consistent monitoring, which went beyond HIV testing, medical practitioners were able to build trust. Services run out of the City Hospital's HIV family clinic were adapted to bridge existing gaps in HIV-affected families' healthcare. Realising that 'these are families that never went for their screening appointments', clinic practitioners designed their intervention to be 'a one-stop shop'.

> [T]hey got the developmental screening and then I would take a clinical history to make sure they were okay, you can imagine the anxiety among a lot of these young women, any snuffle they might be on the phone to you, any contact with chicken pox, you know, they might be on the phone to ask for advice, they didn't go to the GPs. They always bypassed the GPs and they would come straight through to the paediatric clinic.[60]

Taking on the role of GP and providing home visits was often one of the more straightforward adaptations that Mok and her colleagues undertook. Much of the labour involved in meeting the needs of mothers and children affected by HIV was far from usual, especially in the early days. Oral histories from health and social care workers emphasise the way that obstructions created by stigma and the newness of their work often meant workers bridged gaps in services by taking on new roles. Workers also consistently acknowledge some level of courtesy stigma, with their family members fearing for their safety and the general public persistently concerned about contact transmission.[61]

In her oral history testimony, Mok reflected on the ways that she and the health visitor who joined her on home visits had to adapt. Fiona Mitchell, who later became integral to producing the children's books PARC published to meet the emotional and educational needs of HIV-affected children, ended up holding babies during blood lettings alongside her more usual health promotion role. According to Mok, 'she would just hold the baby, squeeze the arm, … whatever was necessary'.[62] Meanwhile Mok, when home visits ran long and she missed the bloods pick-up, found herself acting not only as paediatric HIV specialist and impromptu GP, but as delivery driver, running samples to hospital laboratories.[63] Reflecting on the varied and unpredictable nature of this work, Mok concluded: 'But it was fun. We had a mission. We knew what we were doing.'[64] As the needs of HIV-affected families changed, so too would the means by which Mok met her 'mission'. 'This was the realisation that we might not have enough infected children to keep me [Mok] busy … it dawned on social workers that we might actually have a lot more children affected by HIV rather than infected by HIV.'[65]

The genesis of PARC

Even before anyone realised that the needs of mothers and children might be different from anticipated, the 'innovative nature' of Lothian's response to HIV among mothers and babies meant Mok was in demand. Mok soon began to receive 'requests for information on all aspects of paediatric HIV (not purely clinical) from interested parties within the UK, Europe, and further afield'.[66] In July 1986 a study of mothers and babies with HIV similar to the ECS study was initiated in Zaire (now the Democratic Republic of Congo) involving fellow Edinburgh paediatrician Dr William Cutting. Owing to common interest, the two doctors had extensive contact, but it was not until 1988, when a needs assessment of HIV/AIDS in the Lothian was conducted, that the need for a more formal 'resource centre to handle data and information, to ensure the effective collection and dissemination to those requiring it' around paediatric AIDS was mooted.[67] In February 1991, PARC was officially established using short-term funding from UK children's charity Barnardo's and from the European Community. The centre was based at Edinburgh University's Department of Child Life and Health and received support from the university and LHB but, as was the case for many similar AIDS organisations,

PARC never received long-term funding, instead relying on a variety of small grants, collaborations with other HIV organisations, and the labour of volunteers. Mok and Cutting both acted as directors, but their positions were unpaid.[68]

The explicit aim of PARC was to 'improve the care of children and families with HIV/AIDS by providing information for anyone involved in their welfare'. According to its profile in the Lothian HIV/AIDS newsletter *Meridian*, it achieved this by:

> Publishing and distributing information leaflets
> Responding to telephone, written and personal enquiries
> Organising training courses for groups of child carers
> Holding annual meetings giving a scientific update on HIV in women and children.[69]

To realise these ends, PARC helped facilitate and support the work of other organisations striving to meet the needs of HIV-affected families, enabling charitable and activist organisations to reach wider audiences. For parents affected by HIV, PARC collated together several leaflets written by Dr Mok with the aid of Fiona Mitchell to form 'a parent information pack'. The pack included 'Guidance Notes for Carers'; 'I am HIV+. What Does This Mean for My Child?'; 'My Child is HIV Infected – How Do You Know?'; 'My Child is HIV Infected – Where Do I Go from Here?'; 'My Child is HIV Infected – Signs and Symptoms'; and 'My Child is HIV Infected – What Treatments Are Available?'.[70]

Partially, PARC's leaflets aimed at HIV-positive parents functioned to prepare them for medical encounters inside and outside the home, securing ongoing consent for health interventions such as tests and treatments. However, because of the media's persistent interest in HIV-positive mothers and their babies, the leaflets also worked to redress misinformation and stigma, empowering HIV-affected families and attempting to instil hope. For example, the leaflet 'I am HIV+. What Does This Mean for My Child?' communicated scientific facts in simple terms, but also described one of the 'aims of follow up' as 'To reassure parents where possible that their child has no *signs or symptoms* of HIV infection [emphasis in original]'.[71] The green-and-white leaflet, decorated with teddy bears dressed as doctors, nurses, and patients, explained that '*All babies born to HIV positive mothers will at first be ANTIBODY*

POSITIVE [emphasis in original]', before reassuring parents that 'The city hospital has been following up on babies born to HIV positive mothers since 1985. So far around 10% of these babies are infected with HIV.'[72] After this important framing, the schedule of intense assessment required for babies born to HIV-positive mothers was then given, followed by a list of what such assessments would involve. The daunting future of intense scrutiny was somewhat softened by the leaflet explaining that:

> Approximately 90% of the children being followed up will lose their mother's antibodies around 12–18 months. When this happens we call the child
> *Presumed uninfected.*[73]

The leaflet ends by acknowledging the onerous nature of the medical scrutiny HIV-affected families were under, thanking parents for their cooperation, and reassuring parents that *'all information regarding you and your child will be treated in strictest confidence'* [emphasis in original].[74] Leaflets such as this acted as reference material, allowing HIV-positive mothers to process their diagnosis and the future regime of tests their baby would undergo in their own time, outside the clinical encounter. Within the clinical encounter, they provided a simple script for care practitioners to use, reassuring parents and persuading them to participate in cohort studies. Armed with the knowledge provided by doctors and leaflets such as this, women could more adequately plan for their future, anticipating the likely outcome of their baby being HIV-negative. These interventions had meaningful impacts for HIV-positive and HIV-affected mothers, redressing the hopelessness engendered by the media's representation of HIV. As one adoptive mother of an HIV-positive toddler explained, 'We had a doctor from the Fife Health Board out to counsel us on the virus and realised what the papers were printing on how you catch the virus was very wrong.'[75]

Alongside the creation of published material PARC maintained a large collection of resource materials on a 'wide range of topics relating to the care of children affected by and infected with HIV' and maintained two databases: 'a medical/scientific' database and one collating 'information on organisations and resources'.[76] The creation of these databases and the library of resources was made possible by the centre's keen maintenance of local, national, and international links, allowing it to benefit from, and exchange expertise on, both local and global scales. Thus, while PARC hosted the second International Conference on HIV in Children and Mothers in September 1993, which was opened by Diana, Princess of Wales and attended by over 500 delegates from all over the world, it also maintained more local collaborations. PARC was a member of the National Forum of AIDS and Children (a UK-wide group), the UK NGO AIDS Consortium, the Steering Group on Children and Families Infected and Affected by HIV/AIDS for Children in Scotland, Lothian AIDS Forum's Functional Group on Education and Prevention, and Lothian Information Workers' Network. These regional ties allowed PARC to draw on the expertise of organisations with Lothian knowledge, dealing sensitively with issues around drug use and sexuality by signposting the activist and voluntary organisations best able to help each HIV-affected family.

Though originally envisioned as an information centre, and a way to formalise the signposting and dissemination of HIV/AIDS information which had become informal aspects of Mok and Cuttings' jobs, the project soon took up a more proactive role. PARC began to organise training days aimed at those working with HIV-affected children. The adaptable and evolving biannual course 'Child Care Workers and HIV' was targeted at participants from 'statutory and voluntary sectors' and carers, and hoped to 'promote good practice in the care of children and families affected by HIV, by sharing experiences and expertise, and encouraging a multi-disciplinary approach'.[77] Through its links with regional, national, and international HIV/AIDS organisations, PARC was able to share a wide range of resources and experiences during these training sessions, while signposting other organisations which might be of use to participants and the HIV-affected families they worked with. For example, the one-day workshop PARC held in October 1991 hosted participants who were nurses, doctors, charity workers, council workers, social workers, and play specialists. Attendees were mainly from Edinburgh, Glasgow, London, and Manchester, but also Liverpool, Dundee, Aberdeen, Inverness, Mid Glamorgan, Essex, Carlisle, Carluke, and Wolverhampton.[78] Discussions ranged from confidentiality to bereavement and education, with the Lothian offered up as a case study of best practice.[79]

PARC was also proactive in its approach to meeting the needs of HIV-affected families. After a UK-wide needs assessment of service providers by PARC's coordinator Alison Angus in 1994, the centre sought funding to create resources not just for HIV-positive parents and the guardians of HIV-positive children, but for the HIV-affected children themselves. The UK needs assessment found that the greatest need was for 'information materials which can be used by the increasing numbers of children affected by HIV in families, who are faced with the loss of either, or both, parents'.[80] Three working groups were created to meet children's needs according to age, split between three and seven, eight and twelve, and thirteen and sixteen years, drawing on existing texts PARC had already collected in its library of resources.[81] In part these resources aimed to overcome the reticence of guardians around talking about HIV to their children, filling gaps in the education of HIV-affected children by empowering those that cared for them and the children themselves. Understanding what parents and guardians needed from PARC to facilitate such discussions and to create such targeted resources required the centre to actively assess the needs of mothers and children around HIV disclosure. This meant asking parents, and also children where possible, what they needed. It also meant facilitating the creation of resources by HIV-positive mothers themselves.

PARC, responding to parents' requests 'for books to help them open up' regarding HIV and 'for books that will help them explain how the virus works', produced or facilitated the publication and dissemination of several texts, both factual and fictional.[82] Among these was *It's clinic day*, a picture book by Ruth Stevens, an HIV-positive mother. The book follows a mother and child visiting an HIV clinic modelled on the City Hospital's clinic. By showing encounters with other HIV-affected children, interactions with the paediatrician and health visitor, and delivering simple information about HIV, the book modelled an ideal clinical visit and scripted the parental HIV disclosure for reticent parents.[83] PARC also published a series of picture books written by Fiona Mitchell and illustrated by Mark Mackensie-Smith, which followed Lucy and her mother. *Maybe another day* (1995) follows Lucy as she comes to terms with her mother's illness, realising it is not her fault.

The sequel, *Missing mum* (1996), shows Lucy learning that she will be cared for even when her mother has to attend hospital, and recognising that there are other adults she can trust with her fears. The year 1997 saw the publication of the final two picture books in the series, *Getting to know Sandra* and *Tell me again what happens*, which dealt with respite care and grief.[84] These simple and brightly illustrated books were designed with blank pages so that children could draw their feelings in reaction to the content and the similarities between Lucy's life and their own. Each text concentrated on Lucy's relationship with her mother and other caring adults, offering a textual aid for difficult conversations. PARC also collated an annotated bibliography of books in *What do we tell the children? Books to use with children affected by illness and bereavement* (1996), advising those working with HIV-affected children on how each text could best be deployed and warning adults to supervise children's use of HIV-related materials to prevent unnecessary fear.

In a similar vein to the Lucy series, PARC produced a large activity pack in a brightly illustrated 'attractive' ring-bound folder, *A resource pack for those working with children affected by parental illness* (1997).[85] Again, Mark Mackenzie-Smith provided the illustrations, ensuring a sense of continuity for HIV-affected families who had used the Lucy series. Comprised of short illustrated stories, worksheets, factsheets, and drawing and writing prompts, the pack concentrated on working through thoughts and feelings about the child's present and future. The pack was piloted by the staff and students from several local schools, as well as the hospice Brenda House, the family-focused drug dependency service the Riverside Project, and the children's charity Barnardo's, in an attempt to ensure it was appropriate.

As with the Lucy series, at its heart the pack was a tool for facilitating difficult conversations about HIV-affected family life, created as much for parents as it was for children. As the introduction explained, while parents

> may have difficulties coming to terms with their diagnosis, coping with illness or with fear of stigma ... Children may become confused and fearful from lack of information or misinformation. Their questions may be ignored, answered inadequately or even untruthfully.[86]

While the pack acknowledged that some parents 'refuse to talk or allow others to talk to their children about their illness and its implications for the future', framing this as highly problematic, it also states unequivocally that 'Parents have a right to confidentiality. Children do not have a right to know their parent's diagnosis.'[87] However, because children attended hospital visits, hospices, and had contact with other HIV-related organisations, they were likely to pick up clues about the situation their family was in. Moreover, the pack argued, children 'have the right to participate in decisions concerning their future and to express views on all matters directly affecting them'.[88] The empowering intent of the pack was then clearly stated.

> With help, parents should be the ones to disclose any sensitive information and take responsibility for planning their children's future care. This pack is to help facilitate this process ... to help start a dialogue within the family.[89]

The dialogic nature of the pack was in part encouraged by warnings that children 'should never be expected to attempt the work sheets on their own' but rather with an 'adult sympathetic to the child's needs in attendance', owing to the 'sensitive nature of the materials'.[90] For HIV-affected mothers, the pack offered a variety of sympathetic and carefully scripted routes to talk about HIV, AIDS, and death with their children, easing difficult conversations. Moreover, the very existence of the pack, and similar resources, reassured parents that while difficult, their experiences were not unique. Other HIV-affected families had weathered these difficult conversations and lived to tell the tale (in the form of PARC publications).

Conclusion

The lives of HIV-positive and HIV-affected mothers living in Edinburgh in the last two decades of the twentieth century were shaped by a wide variety of factors. Against a backdrop of media interest in Edinburgh's seemingly unusual demographic spread of HIV infection, mothers' experiences were rendered the stuff of newspaper melodrama and misinformation, engendering feelings of fear and guilt in those newly diagnosed. And yet, living in the 'AIDS capital of Europe' meant access to medical expertise and dedicated paediatric services which emerged relatively quickly at

Edinburgh City Hospital. While other cities' medical responses concentrated on the needs of patients with AIDS, the early recognition of a population living with HIV in Edinburgh created opportunities to differentiate and attend to the specific needs of those living with both HIV and AIDS. However, mothers' emotional and educational needs remained neglected by a national public health response aimed at preventing new infection rather than meeting the needs of those already living with the virus. Moreover, in the scramble to deal with the AIDS crisis, the needs of those affected by HIV, rather than infected with the virus, often remained invisible. This ellipsis has been echoed in the inattention the historiography pays to parenting bonds, and in part accounts for the absence of HIV-affected children from the historiography. Mothers' needs, and the needs of their children, were recognised by those that worked with them, but only received dedicated resources after the acute national crisis was brought under relative control.

PARC encapsulates aspects of the medical, educational, and emotional response to the needs of HIV-affected mothers in Edinburgh. Emerging from medical and social care expertise, PARC's ties with voluntary and activist organisations and its informal beginnings meant it was a reactive organisation which understood the needs of those it served. By analysing PARC's evolution from information hub to publisher, this chapter shines a light on just one organisation, albeit one with important reach, which shaped the lives of HIV-affected mothers in Edinburgh. In doing so, the chapter demonstrates that the recovery of histories which include the experiences of women and children affected by HIV is not only possible, but imperative. While the HIV/AIDS activism of HIV-affected mothers, and those that worked with them, was often low-key and hard to distinguish from the day-to-day of work or survival, it deserves its place in the historical record as much as any act of protest or direct action.

Acknowledgements

I am extremely grateful to my co-editor Janet Weston for her patience and advice, without which this chapter (and this book) would not exist. I am also indebted to the archivists and librarians at the Lothian Health Service Archive whose aid was fundamental and substantial. I would also like to thank Gareth Millward and Martin Moore who read drafts of the chapter, offering sage advice and encouragement. This research was funded by the Wellcome Trust, grant number 219747/Z/19/Z.

Notes

1 This quote is from a collection of the experiences of HIV-affected and HIV-positive Scots compiled by Brid Cullen, a volunteer and later manager of Support on Addiction for Families in Edinburgh (SAFE). It is fairly typical of the assertive testimony which is often found in AIDS anthologies produced by AIDS activists and the voluntary sector. Brid Cullen, *Colours of hope and promise* (Glasgow: Wild Goose Publications, 1999).
2 This quote is demonstrative of the ways newspapers deployed the testimony of the HIV-affected and HIV-positive. Aileen Ballantyne, 'Learning to let mother go', *The Sunday Times*, 22 February 1998.
3 Interview with Jacqueline Mok and Helen Zealley on paediatric care for HIV-affected children and their families, by Louise Williams, 3 July 2018, Acc18/017, Lothian Health Services Archive.
4 Naomi Honigsbaum, *Children and families affected by HIV in Europe: the way forward* (London: The National Children's Bureau, 1994).
5 Hannah J. Elizabeth, '[Re]inventing childhood in the age of AIDS: the representation of HIV positive identities to children and adolescents in Britain, 1983–1997' (unpublished PhD thesis, University of Manchester, 2016).
6 Erving Goffman, *Stigma: notes on the management of spoiled identity* (London: Simon and Schuster, 2009), pp. 30–1; Ann Sutton, Sarah Morton, and David Johnson, 'Key issues in working with children and HIV', in *Children and HIV: supporting children and their families* (Edinburgh: The Stationery Office, 1996), p. 13; R. S. Barbour, 'The implications of HIV/AIDS for a range of workers in the Scottish context', *AIDS Care*, 7.4 (1 October 1995), 521–36. See also Chapter 4 in this collection, on the related idea of 'dirty work'.
7 This chapter is drawn from a much larger research project investigating how HIV-affected families were built and maintained through love, care, and activism between 1981 and 2016. My hope is that publications which address these other familial relationships will follow. https://wellcome.org/grant-funding/people-and-projects/grants-awarded/whats-love-got-do-it-building-and-maintaining-hiv (accessed 5 March 2022).

8 There are of course exceptions, including Virginia Berridge's attention to Scotland and its influence over English policy, in Virginia Berridge, *AIDS in the UK: the making of policy, 1981–1994* (Oxford; New York: Oxford University Press, 1996). This chapter, and the two chapters which precede it, will no doubt soon be joined by a flurry of important publications stemming from recent and ongoing research which seeks to uncover more regional histories of HIV/AIDS in the UK.
9 Matt Cook, '"Archives of feeling": The AIDS crisis in Britain 1987', *History Workshop Journal*, 83.1 (2017), 51–78.
10 Judith Bury, Val Morrison, and Sheena McLachlan, *Working with women and AIDS: medical, social, and counselling issues* (London: Psychology Press, 1992).
11 It is worth noting that other cities in and beyond Europe also earned this unhappy accolade, as discussed in the Introduction to this collection. Similar high infection rates among intravenous drug users in Switzerland earned Berne the same title, for example. Christine Toomey, 'Drug-haunted Berne makes fixing official', *The Sunday Times*, 2 July 1989, p. 20; Ballantyne, 'Learning to let mother go'.
12 Sheila M. Burns, Raymond P. Brettle, Sheila M. Gore, John F. Peutherer, and J. Roy Robertson, 'The epidemiology of HIV infection in Edinburgh related to the injecting of drugs: an historical perspective and new insight regarding the past incidence of HIV infection derived from retrospective HIV antibody testing of stored samples of serum', *Journal of Infection*, 32.1 (1996), 53–62.
13 J. R. Robertson, A. B. Bucknall, P. D. Welsby, J. J. Roberts, J. M. Inglis, J. F. Peutherer, et al., 'Epidemic of AIDS related virus (HTLV-III/LAV) infection among intravenous drug abusers', *British Medical Journal (Clinical Research Ed.)*, 292.6519 (1986), 527–9.
14 Bury, Morrison, and McLachlan, *Working with women and AIDS*, pp. 10–12.
15 *Ibid*.
16 *Ibid*.
17 Naomi Honigsbaum, *HIV, AIDS and children: a cause for concern* (London: National Children's Bureau, 1991), p. 8.
18 Alex Mold, 'Just say know: drug education and its publics in 1980s Britain', *The International Journal on Drug Policy*, 88 (2021), 103029.
19 Margaret Harker, 'Councils urged: do more in AIDS fight', *Edinburgh Evening News*, 8 August 1988, GD1/12/2/3 (313) AIDS press cuttings, Lothian Health Services Archive.
20 John Street, 'British government policy on AIDS: learning not to die of ignorance', *Parliamentary Affairs*, 41.4 (1988): 490–507; Colin Moore, 'Communicating prevention: the Scottish experience of health

education in the AIDS epidemic, 1981–1996' (unpublished master's thesis, Glasgow, University of Strathclyde, 2019), pp. 55–7.
21 Anne Barrowclough and Marie Scott, 'My guilt when they said I'd given my baby AIDS', *Daily Mail*, 27 October 1986, p. 12.
22 See, for example, William Daniels, 'Secret AIDS watch on a mother and baby', *Daily Mirror*, 21 December 1984, p. 2; Jill Palmer, 'AIDS baby nightmare: mum must wait to see if her baby will live', *Daily Mirror*, 20 February 1985, pp. 1–2; Jill Palmer, 'Wife get AIDS from husband's affair: death risk forces mum-to-be to have an abortion', *Daily Mirror*, 23 October 1986, p. 7; William Davies, 'Double curse of the aids plague city: the drugs were bad enough… now the addicts' needles are creating a horror on a unique scale behind Edinburgh's elegant façade', *Daily Mail*, 11 April 1986, p. 6.
23 Steven F. Kruger, *AIDS narratives: gender, sexuality, fiction and science*, 1st edn (New York: Routledge, 1997), p. 81; Elizabeth, '[Re]inventing childhood in the age of AIDS', pp. 48–9.
24 *Ibid.*
25 Kruger, *AIDS narratives*, pp. 75–6; Elizabeth, '[Re]inventing childhood in the age of AIDS', pp. 48–9.
26 Kruger, *AIDS narratives*, pp. 73–9.
27 Barrowclough and Scott, 'My guilt'.
28 *Ibid.*
29 *Ibid.*
30 C. McCarthy and P. D. Welsby, 'Edinburgh – the AIDS capital of Europe?', *Scottish Medical Journal*, 48.1 (2003), 3–5.
31 Barrowclough and Scott, 'My guilt'.
32 *Ibid.*
33 *Ibid.*
34 *Ibid.* For an in-depth look at nursing practices around HIV/AIDS, see Chapter 4 in this volume.
35 Centers of Disease Control, 'Current trends acquired immunodeficiency syndrome (AIDS) update – United States', *Morbidity and Mortality Weekly Report*, 32.24 (1983), 309–11.
36 Barrowclough and Scott, 'My guilt'.
37 *Ibid.*
38 *Ibid.*
39 Similar histories of integrated HIV/AIDS networks could be told by looking at the emergence of LGBTQ responses to HIV/AIDS in Edinburgh. Much of this history is yet to be written, but see, for health education and policy response, Moore, 'Communicating prevention'; Helen Coyle, 'A tale of one city: a history of HIV/AIDS policy-making in Edinburgh, 1982–1994' (unpublished PhD thesis, University of Edinburgh, 2008).

40 Zealley and Mok were interviewed together by Louise Williams of the Lothian Health Service Archive (LHSA) in 2018. As former colleagues, the conversation flowed freely and informally, with the two joking together and reminding one another of their past experiences with little input from Williams.
41 Jacqueline Mok and Sarah Cooper, 'The needs of children whose mothers have HIV infection', *Archives of Disease in Childhood*, 77.6 (1997), 483–7.
42 Williams, interview with Mok and Zealley on paediatric care.
43 *Ibid.*
44 *Ibid.*
45 Coyle, 'A tale of one city', pp. 118–20.
46 Cullen, *Colours of hope and promise*, p. 101.
47 Williams, interview with Mok and Zealley on paediatric care.
48 Cullen, *Colours of hope and promise*, pp. 101–6.
49 Williams, interview with Mok and Zealley on paediatric care.
50 Jacqueline Mok, R. A. Hague, P. L. Yap, F. D. Hargreaves, J. M. Inglis, J. M. Whitelaw, C. M. Steel, O. B. Eden, S. Rebus, J. F. Peutherer, 'Vertical transmission of HIV: a prospective study', *Archives of Disease in Childhood*, 64.8 (1989), 1140–5.
51 Jacqueline Mok and Fiona Mitchell, 'Communicating with parents and children about medical and nursing procedures', in *Children and HIV: supporting children and their families*, ed. by Sarah Morton and David Johnson (Edinburgh: Children in Scotland, 1996), p. 49.
52 *Ibid.*
53 The European Collaborative Study, 'Mother-to-child transmission of HIV infection: the European Collaborative Study', *The Lancet*, 2.8619 (1988), 1039–43.
54 Williams, interview with Mok and Zealley on paediatric care.
55 *Ibid.*
56 *Ibid.*
57 Mok and Cooper, 'The needs of children whose mothers have HIV infection', p. 483.
58 Honigsbaum, *HIV, AIDS and children*, p. 130.
59 Williams, interview with Mok and Zealley on paediatric care.
60 *Ibid.*
61 Cullen, *Colours of hope and promise*, pp. 78–86.
62 Williams, interview with Mok and Zealley on paediatric care.
63 *Ibid.*
64 *Ibid.*
65 *Ibid.*
66 'Paediatric AIDS Resource Centre (PARC)', *Meridian*, July 1994, GD/22/8/1, Lothian Health Services Archive.

67 *Ibid.*
68 *Ibid.*
69 *Ibid.*
70 *Ibid.*
71 PARC, 'I am HIV+. What Does This Mean for My Child?' (Edinburgh: PARC, 1991).
72 *Ibid.*
73 *Ibid.*, emphasis in original.
74 *Ibid.*
75 Extract from AIDS Bulletin, June 1988, published by Social Work Service Group, Scottish Education Department, quoted in Naomi Honigsbaum, *Living and working with HIV: training guidance for staff in the personal social services* (London: Central Council For Education and Training in Social Work, 1989), p. 63.
76 'Paediatric AIDS Resource Centre (PARC)', *Meridian*, July 1994, GD/22/8/1, Lothian Health Services Archive.
77 *Ibid.*
78 Jaqueline Mok, William A. M. Cutting, Lesley Reid, Joy Barlow, 'Child care workers and HIV' (Edinburgh: PARC, 1991), LHB45/1/4/9 (1:2) & LHB45/1/4/9 (2:2), Lothian Health Services Archive.
79 *Ibid.*
80 'Paediatric AIDS Resource Centre (PARC)', *Meridian*, July 1994, GD/22/8/1, Lothian Health Services Archive.
81 *Ibid.*
82 Kerstin B. Phillips, *What do we tell the children? Books to use with children affected by illness and bereavement* (Edinburgh: PARC, 1996).
83 Elizabeth, '[Re]inventing childhood in the age of AIDS', pp. 214–32.
84 Fiona Mitchell and Mark Mackenzie-Smith, *Tell me again what happens* (Edinburgh: PARC, 1997); Fiona Mitchell and Mark Mackenzie-Smith, *Getting to know Sandra* (Edinburgh: PARC, 1997).
85 PARC Working Group, *Activity pack: a resource pack for those working with children affected by parental illness* (Edinburgh: PARC, 1997).
86 *Ibid.*
87 *Ibid.*
88 *Ibid.*
89 *Ibid.*
90 *Ibid.*

7

The European HIV/AIDS Archive: building a queer counter-memory

Agata Dziuban, Eugen Januschke, Ulrike Klöppel, Todd Sekuler, and Justyna Struzik

If you noticed, when you ask me about the history of AIDS... I can talk forever, because there are very few people with whom I share that. The majority of them have died. And even if I have new friends from a younger generation... Sometimes I feel like I don't wanna put the burden of this history on someone by telling them. I don't wanna tell the young people who are starting to work in the HIV field unless they wanna know, because they must have the freedom and the space to develop their own ideas, right? And... well, I'm happy to talk to you and share some information, as many people just simply don't want to know. They don't want to know. When I tell, told my parents what I'm doing, they said, 'And is anybody listening to you?' So I decided, well, maybe I do not go into much detail about my work and I give a list of when I'm at home or not at home, you know? And so with friends, in 1997... people died, that year I lost something like forty or fifty colleagues. When I told this, a friend, the reaction was, 'Why didn't they take the new treatments?' You see how difficult it is to talk about your experiences to someone who is not familiar with the field and who doesn't really want to be involved? A very good friend of mine has lost a brother, who was an injecting drug user, to AIDS. You know, understanding goes without words. She knows why I'm doing it and she has been through this on a very personal level. But many people just simply say, 'Oh, is it still a problem?' ... You are isolated in a way, you know? ... Sometimes you don't know where to go with all your memories or impressions, losses, grief, fun situations you have seen. And that is, that is something, which I think an oral history project should capture. That's why I allowed the filming.[1]

The European HIV/AIDS Archive 193

Mobilising a queer theoretical framework, by which we mean embracing unhappiness, ephemerality, and instability, this chapter attempts to put into words some of what goes 'without words' in the understandings and narrations of engagements with the HIV/AIDS epidemic. It explores the tensions, documented in audio, video, and language, between a need to speak and the experience or anticipation of being met with indifference or non-comprehension. The above excerpt from an interview with Stephen Dressler, co-founder of the European AIDS Treatment Group (EATG), the longest existing network of individuals united in responding to the continued impact of the epidemic from across the Europe region, is part of the newly launched European HIV/AIDS Archive that provides the material for the focus of this chapter. In this extract, Stephen problematises his own position as a narrator of history, as a veteran and long-term activist who has witnessed the horrors of mass AIDS-related deaths in the 1980s and 1990s, vis-à-vis new generations of HIV/AIDS activists who have often only recently come to be engaged in the field, and who are faced with unique challenges and different ways of thinking and acting in response to the epidemic. Prompted by this excerpt, and using this chapter to reflect on the process of archiving oral histories, we unravel various challenges and tensions that lie at the heart of remembering, narrating, and archiving the HIV/AIDS epidemic in the broader European region.

The European HIV/AIDS Archive (EHAA) is an online collection of narratives of the past, present, and imagined futures of the HIV/AIDS epidemic in the European region.[2] We see the archive as *living* because it is meant to enhance understanding of HIV/AIDS history, stimulate new readings, and inspire additional oral history work on the topic.[3] It brings together a wide range of oral history interviews – personal accounts of living with and responding to HIV/AIDS – complemented by links to policy documents and artworks that allow us to immerse ourselves in the complex history of the epidemic in Europe. The archive opens a space to preserve and share memories of living with or in times of HIV/AIDS. At the heart of the collection are the narratives of people living with the virus, of representatives of communities most affected by it, and of advocates and activists, politicians and policy-makers, healthcare workers, employees of aid organisations, and artists.

The EHAA complements and expands upon the predominantly nationally focused HIV/AIDS archives that already exist in selected European countries.[4] Simultaneously, it builds on a conviction that the history of the epidemic in the European region has not been adequately recorded, while acknowledging that it can never be recorded completely. While most analyses and cultural representations of activist engagements with HIV/AIDS and political responses to the spread of the virus have focused on the USA[5] and, less frequently, on selected countries of the Global South,[6] attention has more rarely been directed towards the unfolding of the epidemic in different parts of Europe,[7] especially Eastern, Southern, or Central Europe. It was also not uncommon as we were developing this archive to discover that valuable personal and institutional materials and stories had been destroyed (due to floods, such as with parts of the World Health Organization-Europe and EATG archives), abandoned (as activists moved houses, countries, or continents), or otherwise lost. In those contexts where HIV/AIDS narratives have already been partially preserved, we felt that there was a need to render these histories more complex, to account for the stories of groups of persons, such as migrants, sex workers, people who use drugs, prisoners, and members of religious communities, whose perspectives, lived experiences, and struggles in the context of HIV/AIDS have often been rendered singular, marginalised, or forgotten.[8]

We hope that the framing and existence of this archive will enable reflection, using this and other collections, to better understand the histories of HIV/AIDS and, generally, the politics of health and the imagined futurities of existence in the European region. With the EHAA, we aim to commemorate, document, and learn from activist, civil society, and other policy-maker efforts in the field of HIV/AIDS, or in closely related areas, such as in sex work, drug policy, LGBTQI+ rights, or the health and legal status of migrants or prisoners. We believe that it can also illustrate how HIV/AIDS activism has been built upon and led to unique forms of solidarity, empowerment, political intervention, and organising, and suggest what sought-after futures reveal about the perceived possibilities and constraints of the present. As a social and political practice, the archive has been developed to help work through the trauma of loss and social discrimination – a process that can often be met with only limited understanding by friends and family members, as the opening interview excerpt illustrates.[9] The archive also documents innovations, tensions, and inconsistencies in engaging with the epidemic, up to the present. By creating a space to share, compare, and gather these stories, the EHAA offers a living memory of recent and contemporary HIV/AIDS history in the twenty-first century.

In all of these dimensions, the EHAA contributes to queer memory work as a necessary revision of public remembrance and current perceptions of the epidemic, and, at the same time, as a source of inspiration for future activism. Explicitly deviating from an investment in offspring as route for the transmission of memory, the EHAA joins other queer archival work that has 'been fashioned as agentic sites for passing on and handing down queer history'.[10] In this chapter we discuss these arguments in more detail, after we first present a brief overview of the archive's structure.

The archive

The EHAA is a searchable online collection of testimonies addressing the history and unfolding present of individual, social, and political responses to HIV/AIDS in Europe. A limited number of interviews are available to view on-site only; the majority can either be downloaded or viewed online. The archive has been developed as a space to preserve memories of living with the virus, and of activist and civil society engagements and HIV/AIDS policies in Europe, with an aim to share stories and learn from a variety of voices and experiences. The EHAA consists primarily of video- and audio-recorded oral history interviews – a method intentionally selected to grasp the unfolding of historical events and processes from the first-hand individual and personal perspectives of those whose voices are often excluded from usual archival strategies and dominant narratives.[11] Oral histories enable a lively and multi-perspective memory. Topics include everyday life with HIV and AIDS, self-help, activism, sex work, drugs, migration, refugees, prisons, LGBTQI+ rights, and queer politics. The oral history interviews are supplemented by digitised photos, grey literature, policy documents, and documentation of activist interventions and engagements with the epidemic.

Inspired by different efforts to account for and preserve the lived experiences of the HIV/AIDS epidemic worldwide, and especially the online archive of the ACT UP Oral History Project,[12] the EHAA oral history archive initiative dates back to the AIDS History into Museums Working Group (AKAIM) of the German AIDS Service Organisation (Deutsche AIDS-Hilfe e.V.). Within AKAIM, a subgroup came together in 2015 with the aim of interviewing contemporary witnesses and setting up an oral history archive. In cooperation with this group, the idea was further developed within two research projects: 'Disentangling European HIV/AIDS Policies: Activism, Citizenship and Health' (EUROPACH) and 'Don't Criminalize Passion! The AIDS Crisis and Political Mobilization in the 1980s and Early 1990s in Germany'. The EUROPACH project, a collaboration between Humboldt-Universität zu Berlin, Jagiellonian University, Goldsmiths, University of London, the University of Basel, and a great number of activist groups and non-governmental organisations, explores the practices of HIV/AIDS policy development, negotiation, and contestation in Germany, Poland, Turkey, the UK, and at the European level. While the research topic for certain EUROPACH researchers was focused on a specific field of HIV/AIDS activism, such as harm reduction in prisons and prisoners' rights in Germany, other researchers investigated a multitude of grassroots responses to HIV/AIDS to reconstruct histories of activism as broadly as possible. The second project, '"Don't Criminalize Passion!"', which was based at the Humboldt-Universität zu Berlin, investigates the formation of the AIDS movement during the 1980s and early 1990s in the Federal Republic of Germany. These two projects had different research foci, but also complemented each other well. Oral history interviews carried out by AKAIM and both of these subsequent research projects will be included in the EHAA. As all three projects were inspired by a queer theoretical approach, this has had an impact on the development of the EHAA. In the following sections, we will reconstruct this approach from the perspective of the two contributing research groups, as a contribution to a queer counter-memory.

Collection holdings

The EHAA collection consists mainly of video interviews and, secondarily, of audio interviews or interview transcripts. By interviews we also mean conversations with multiple interview partners, including focus groups and witness seminars.[13] Interviews constituting the EHAA are heterogeneous in other ways, as each narrative is shaped by the lived experiences and particularities of the biographical trajectories of each interview partner. As of early 2022, approximately seventy such interviews form the basis of the collection and at least thirty more will be uploaded in the near future. As we continue to develop plans of collaboration with HIV-related researchers and activists from across the region, it is our hope that the EHAA will be continuously expanded with the addition of interviews from other initiatives and projects.

As much as possible, additional resources, transcripts, curricula vitae, personal documents belonging to the interviewees, and personal photos are also included in the collection. Other digital materials, such as photo documentation, recordings of performances, policy documents, or talks, can also be included in the collection if copyrights or licences permit. So far, given the national foci of the participating projects, interviews have been conducted in Polish, Turkish, English, German, and Russian. Although several Turkish interviews have already been translated into German for a German-language oral history publication on HIV/AIDS activism in Turkey,[14] most other interviews are only available in the original interview language. That being said, translations of transcripts into other languages are planned but will ultimately depend on resource availability.

The collected interviews address many different topics, including, for example, emotions within political mobilisation, the heterogeneity of the HIV/AIDS movement, and varied positions of power and the consequent tensions between actors. In terms of content, the interview collection can be characterised by the following three dimensions, which were also among the meta-data used to order archive entries. First, through the *time period* of interviewees' engagements with HIV/AIDS, which range from the early 1980s to the present. At times, the oral histories also trace activist narratives back to even earlier dates and collectivising movements. Second, the interviews can be grouped by the different – and oftentimes flexible – *positionalities* of those providing their narratives. The interview partners come from activism, self-help structures, non-governmental organisations (NGOs), government bodies and parties, civil society, the biomedical sciences, and fields of social and care work, all fields of activity that often overlap and merge with one another during an interviewee's lifetime. Some of the interviewees were first activists, then NGO staff members, and finally politicians or government officials. One interviewee was a doctor who became active in lobbying, promoting, and implementing drug substitution; another was initially involved in a sex worker organisation dealing with HIV/AIDS and later wrote crime novels. Among the interviewees are people who describe themselves as gay, lesbian, non-binary, woman living with HIV, refugee, trans person, former prisoner, migrant, feminist, person of colour, religious person, sex worker, and person who uses drugs – to name just a few self-ascribed labels, which of course also intersect for various interviewees.

Third, the interview collection can be sorted based on the *topics discussed* by interview partners. The interviews cover a wide range of topics including drug use and harm reduction, prisons and prisoners' rights, empowerment, loss, death and collective mourning, public sex, lesbian safer-sex porn, gender and sexual identity, the women's health movement, trans issues, autonomous sex worker and migrant organisations, forced testing of prisoners and refugees, human rights instruments, children with HIV/AIDS, haemophilia, experiences of social inequality and discrimination, criminalisation and law enforcement, professionalisation, transnational relations, sexually transmitted infections, biopharmaceuticals and the pharmaceutical industry, funding, research, prevention, testing policies, palliative care, and art.

Taken together, these three dimensions exhibit the richness of the collection. Potential users of the EHAA can select entries based on these criteria to search for materials that reflect their own interests or respond to their specific questions.

Infrastructure and usage of interviews

With its media repository, Humboldt-Universität zu Berlin offers the technical infrastructure for storing, managing, and making accessible the digital oral history interviews and other contemporary testimonies and digitised documents that make up the EHAA. The media repository is a digital asset management system. It enables the permanent storage and persistent identification of the collection's objects via unique Digital Object Identifiers (DOIs), metadata that are freely searchable online, the streaming or downloading of specific objects, and differentiated public access to the archival materials. To facilitate use of the archive, topics have been turned into keywords, categories, and other metadata, which make it easier to search the archive's holdings. Other metadata include language, country, discussed events, organisations and institutions, or the names of interviewees (if they have consented to our including them). The metadata is available in English by default but, depending on time and resources, we intend to make metadata available in at least German, Polish, and Turkish as well.

Interviews might be used for a number of purposes, such as teaching, exhibitions, and research or analyses by activists, policy-makers, or scholars in the humanities or social sciences. The interviews have already been at the focus of a EUROPACH concluding exhibition entitled *HIVstories: Living Politics*,[15] which travelled to gallery and museum spaces in Berlin, Warsaw, and Istanbul. In addition, publications from both research projects based on the archived materials are forthcoming. Most of the interviews are freely accessible online, but some can only be viewed on-site in the university library upon request. Users are only permitted to view the latter holdings if they agree to anonymise any of the viewed materials, in accordance with the wishes of the interviewees.

Queer counter-memory

For us, the potential of the EHAA lies in the idea of contributing to a queer counter-memory. It forms a rich source of materials for queer memory work that intervenes into public perceptions of the HIV/AIDS epidemic and opens possibilities for the political struggles of activists today. Guided by a queer intersectional approach, which is sensitive to the entwinements of multiple power relations, non-hegemonic discourses and practices, the fragility of social categorisations – often taken for granted – and the multidimensionality of experiences and lives, we have worked to assemble a diversity of narratives to make up the initial foundation of the archive. This approach also informed the focus of interview questions, which sought to grasp various, fluid, dissonant, and ambivalent feelings of belonging to social movements,[16] and the impact of multiple structural issues on the lives, strategies, and practices of interview partners. With the same methodological lens, we created an archive inventory to make the collection's resources accessible to queer and intersectional readings.

In the next section, we propose reflections on the notions of 'queer memory' and 'queering the archive' that inspired our approach. These considerations are not meant to define the EHAA as an archive that is somehow queer, but are instead meant to be stimuli for discussion on the queer theoretical positioning of the archive's collections, which follows from the different perspectives of the three projects that played a decisive role in its development. For this reason, we do not attempt to smooth out tensions in the perspectives and meanings of what constitutes queer among the variously positioned projects, activists, researchers, and interview partners. If one approach is to identify the political culmination of queer in some kind of reference to non-heteronormative life worlds, then there is also a justification for an understanding of queer as 'taking queer forms of thought out into non-queer worlds of practices and things'.[17] In this respect, our reflections are characterised by meandering tensions and other complex relationships between non-heteronormative and generally non-hegemonic life worlds and queer theoretical forms of thought.

Between queer utopian memory and the unhappy archive

Utopia, writes José Esteban Muñoz, 'permits us to conceptualize new worlds and realities that are not irrevocably constrained by the HIV/AIDS pandemic and institutionalized state homophobia. More importantly, utopia offers us a critique of the present, of what is, by casting a picture of what can and perhaps will be.'[18] Muñoz's arguments for the necessity of a queer utopian memory that inspires a 'political desire' to transform the present has contributed to a rich discussion about queer memory and archival work.[19] Conversations with our interviewees inspire such 'utopian longings'[20] about experiences of solidarity and empowerment in self-help-groups, about the importance of community meeting places such as cafés, clubs, switchboards, cruising areas, drug scenes, sex work venues, or community-led drop-ins, about community events like annual meetings of people living with HIV/AIDS as feel-good resources, or about pangs of desire in activists' meetings.

On the other hand, Heather Love has warned against idealised visions of the past that ignore 'the wounds, the switchbacks, and the false starts'.[21] She urges to shift the 'focus on the negative affects – the need, the aversion, and the longing – that characterize the relation between past and present'.[22] Applying the same perspectival twist, Sara Ahmed calls for an 'unhappy archive' that counters the recent trend towards the social integration and normalisation of LGBTQI+ persons, and the correlating paradigm of a history of progress.[23] Indeed, the oral histories of crises assembled in the EHAA – crises of, for example, AIDS, poverty, rights violations, and criminalisation – are infused with memories and ongoing conditions of injury and vulnerability. Yet, they complicate and go beyond the dualistic notions of happiness and unhappiness, failure and success, progress and backlash. Discussions about community feelings (feelings about community and feelings shared across communities) with our interview partners provide insights into the coexistence of the different affective dimensions of experiences: memories of the power of community feeling that are intertwined with memories of peer pressure, ignorance, internal tensions, negotiations and conflicts, or processes of disidentification and exclusion. The complexity of accounts of the past from interview partners demonstrates how utopian and negative community feelings are oftentimes closely knitted together.

Two examples illustrate this need to complicate the binary of happiness and unhappiness, failure and success, and progress and backlash. First, selected materials from the archive communicate an ongoing feeling of frustration due to stagnation and a never-ending sense of struggle in the face of a constantly changing horizon of possibilities.[24] In certain regions and cities of Poland, for example, recently introduced 'LGBT free-zones', smear campaigns against harm-reduction activists and organisations, attempts to criminalise sex education, and everyday 'state' homophobia contribute to a sense of precarity. As described by several interview partners, this further shapes forms of vulnerability in relation to HIV/AIDS. While some experience this as a backlash, others describe it as a continuity of the same state-sponsored violence. In both instances, these political shifts have provoked self-organising and fierce protests that reveal a striving towards utopian futures despite a sense of hopelessness and fatalism, or what Lauren Berlant has productively termed 'cruel optimism'.[25] From this perspective, even a queer desire to move beyond the binary of progress and backlash might be further queered, in that it presumes that an agreed-upon history of progress already exists in the broader cultural imaginary.

A second example, taken from an interview with an activist from Scotland, also concerns the coexistence of contradicting temporalities of social and political change. While many in the gay community applauded the legalisation of gay marriage and other perceived symptoms of enhanced equality and integration in Scotland in the 2010s, one interviewee described the contemporaneous introduction of new policies and policing strategies targeting men who have sex with men, which included police raids on saunas and the confiscation of condoms. These recent police interventions were described in the interview as though they were moving Scotland back in time to the early 1980s – that is, to a time when public health interventions were hampered by harsh law enforcement strategies and rights violations. Complicating the binary of change and transformation as defined by either success or failure, this coexistence of lived senses of progress and regress in a particular context reveals temporalities of social and political change as contradictory, unstable, and conditional. The oral history collection of the EHAA presents a range of heterogeneous, context-dependent stories of partial empowerment and bad feelings, failures and successes, progress and regress. Thus, it allows users of the archive to problematise these notions by showing their precariousness, ambiguities, and changeability. Instead of providing psychological reassurance from history, this archive enables, as Tavia Nyong'o has suggested with regard to queer archives in general, a 'radical defamiliarization of knowledge' about the AIDS crisis.[26]

Ephemera as evidence

Another guiding reflection during the construction of the archive has been Esteban Muñoz's discussion of the queer meaning of the ephemeral in his essay *Ephemera as evidence*.[27] He argues that queer worlds were often hidden and queer battles were mostly fought in secret, which is why their traces had to be blurred as much as possible. This concealment of queer practices is caused by state violence and pressures from the prevailing (hetero-)normative culture, which is reinforced by the exclusionary practices of public archives: from the destruction of files by descendants or archives themselves (for example, because they classify files as not worthy of archiving) to archival classification systems, which make the remaining traces untraceable.[28] Finding such precarious remnants often requires a sensitivity to hidden, indirect, ephemeral, and transient clues, based on queer and other non-normative experiences.[29] Similarly, Avery Gordon describes 'other utopianism' as a quest for the 'illegible, illegitimate, or trivialized forms of escape, resistance, opposition, and alternative ways of life'.[30] This attention to the ephemeral, illegible, and illegitimate necessitates a queer reading – a speculative reading informed by non-normative experiences and a desire for what items or stories could mean or could have meant for marginalised persons and communities.[31] From our point of view, oral history is most suitable for tracing such precarious hints of queer life worlds and struggles, both during the interview itself and in the later interpretation of the narrative. Audio and video recordings further help to make these hints audible and visible through pauses, intonation, and body language.

Two examples will help to illustrate what this could mean, one from 'Don't Criminalize Passion!' and another from the EUROPACH project. In the first example, one interviewee spoke about a dance marathon in Nuremberg in 1994 that engaged with the ongoing AIDS crisis and AIDS-related loss of lives. For the participants of the event, he said, this was a 'key moment'. Despite the importance of the event as described by our interview partner, there is nothing to be found about it in existing archives. While telling the story, the interviewee burst into tears several times. Yet, he hardly ever talked about personal experiences of loss and grief.[32] We, as interviewers (two persons with different backgrounds, in fact), in turn reacted with alarm and emotion, even though the events narrated were, soberly considered, not dramatic in themselves, even more so since they happened a long time ago. But the way the narrator expressed himself echoed with our embodied emotional practices of collective grief and trauma awareness, which served as a compass to dive deeper into details of the story, both during the interview by interacting with the interviewee and by interpreting it later on.[33] The interviewee explicitly named moments of collective grief, and his outburst of tears made the emotional intensity of the dance marathon palpable. On one hand, there was hardly anything to be learned about the interviewee's *individual* confrontation with the fear of dying and mourning for the dead. Still, his narrative offered breaks and emotional turns that might be read as traumatic effects that dynamise connections between collective and individual grief. At the same time, though, as in a tilted mirror, it is possible to read the interview sequence as provoked by a fundamental disjunction between collective and individual grief, with the latter playing no psychodynamic role at all in the narrative.

Evidence is also made precarious, and reduced to traces that risk becoming invisible, by the privileging of queer understood primarily through the lens of sexuality. As such, the concealment of non-normative practices is caused not only by the pressures of the prevailing (hetero-)normative culture, but by the dominance of gay lives and loss in the imagined and imaginable necropolitical landscape of the epidemic.[34] While working towards developing the archive, we could not only see the complex entanglements of individual and collective grief, but also situate those entanglements in the political and social realities of (un)mournability that selectively grant communities the right to be grieved and grieving.[35] For example, one interviewee narrated the moment when she came to realise that her own life and the lives of her community members – people who use drugs and are living with HIV and AIDS – were not constructed as worthy of recognition and commemoration in the same ways as other non-normative lives, even as experienced by herself and others in her community. This realisation occurred during a visit to a community space for people living with HIV/AIDS in London where she participated in the much-valued collective mourning of yet another gay male friend who had died of complications related to the virus. While talking to another friend whose husband, a person who injected drugs, had also died of AIDS but whose death went all but unacknowledged by her friends and broader communities, she realised that it did not even cross her mind to commemorate the death of her friends who used drugs. This realisation brought her into drug users' rights activism and contributed to the development of the first lifestyle magazine for people who use drugs in the UK, *Black Poppy*, also among the first in Europe.

What her narrative underscores is the fragility and conditionality that lies behind the individual and collective possibility to narrate the epidemic, to engage in recognition struggles,[36] or even to mourn. In the early days of the epidemic, before effective treatment was available and when death was taking its heaviest toll in those communities most vulnerable to HIV/AIDS, the opportunity to confront the fact of someone's death and mourn it individually or collectively could be seen as one of the very few possibilities to make visible, account for, and narrate non-normative lives and experiences. The very construction of someone's (and your own) life as worthy of being acknowledged is a precondition for it to be remembered and preserved in an archive. Thus, the lives and deaths of some were, and still can be, seen as ephemera in the archive of mourning, coming to light only if mediated by the stories of others.

Destabilising categories

The archive has demanded the development of strategies that help us to navigate through materials, make connections across a multiplicity of sources, and build bridges between dissimilar moments, experiences, and localities. As mentioned above, one such strategy has been the construction and application of metadata: a rich web of categories that label interviews and other sources based on the themes, events, organisations, and self-ascribed identities they include. Categories are, however, always already situated in existing webs of meaning and understandings of reality, which are not necessarily translatable across and within different localities, temporalities, and communities.[37] As part of these projects, we explore in this section the intrinsic instability, historical changeability, and contextuality of categories put to use to describe lived experiences, positionalities, and forms of collective and self-identification. To this end, we show how the collected materials exceed the very categories that have been developed from the materials themselves.

Exemplary of such malleability, tension, and instability is the category 'queer', which was used by several interviewed activists as a self-definition and also as a form of coalitional politics, not only against heteronormativity, but also against intersecting norms of respectability, ableism, classism, or racism. Yet this notion and its semantic fields are alien to, and viewed with scepticism or differently understood by, a great variety of possible and actual interviewees. This is related to its perceived origins as an initially 'Western' concept of critical practice or identification, and also the politics of its usage, where some see it as only superficially or problematically including their perspectives, experiences, and communities. It is also often used in its original English version and not translated into other languages. Even for some of the interviewed older gay AIDS activists from Western Europe, queer was not embraced either as a self-definition or as a label of political practice. And yet these same interviewees offered us enthusiastic descriptions of political coalitions with lesbians, sex workers, or persons who use drugs, with focused actions on cross-identity and intersectional marginalisation processes: an approach that exceeds identity-based activism, which can be grasped analytically as 'queer' even if it was not explicitly described or developed as such in the interviews.[38]

For instance, a slogan from a big demonstration in July 1988 in Frankfurt against repressive AIDS politics expressed this new form of coalitional politics: 'Solidarity of the Unreasonable'. As an intersectional intervention, narratives of this event resembled the coalition work of ACT UP New York that Cathy J. Cohen described as queer 'transformative politics'.[39]

Assigning 'queer' as metadata to those interviews, so as to account for discussions about intersectional, coalitional politics, is meant to facilitate research on these queer elements of the archive and of HIV/AIDS activism in Europe, and also, in our practice of assigning metadata to these materials, on the construction of the term queer at this particular historical juncture.

To the extent that the meanings and uses of 'queer' vary considerably across the broader European region, critical reflection about the categories used in the archive also take on a geopolitical dimension. These geopolitical tensions in the terminology of applied metadata are further evidenced by the question of the EHAA's scope, regions, and boundaries. This is already manifest in the archive's title, in which we use 'Europe' as a frame of reference for documenting and analysing engagements with the epidemic. While it must be acknowledged that the primarily European focus of the EHAA only adds to the need to 'provincialise' Europe in future archiving of the epidemic globally,[40] its framing nonetheless also destabilises the cohesion and meaning of Europe in three important ways.

First, the focal countries of the projects that constitute the archive's initial foundation push up against popular framings of Europe. In particular, they centre countries along the borders of what is commonly termed 'Western Europe', even as the precise meaning of what constitutes the 'West' varies based on the labelling individual, network, organisation, or governing body. Inspired by postcolonial scholarship, Robert Kulpa and Joanna Mizielińska thus refer to the localities of Central and Eastern Europe (CEE) as the 'contemporary peripheries': ' "European enough" (geographically), "yet not enough advanced" to become "Western" (temporally)'.[41] Jill Owczarzak has similarly written that CEE is often grasped as 'the West's intermediary "Other", neither fully civilized nor fully savage'.[42] In this dynamic, postsocialist societies, according to Rasa Navickaité, are always going to be 'just an imitation of what has already happened in the West'.[43] Indeed, conducting interviews in different parts of Europe helped us to critically reflect on these 'East'/'West' and 'North'/'South' divisions as malleable, in that they are constructed relationally and variably across time and space, and also as generative, in that they involve shaping practices, political strategies, and forms of individual and collective subjectivities.

Second, while the archive has an initial focus on only four particular countries, the fifth transnational 'European' level at which materials were gathered has enabled the collection of stories that extend from Western Europe into the region commonly referred to as Eastern Europe and Central Asia (EECA). The EHAA includes, for example, the voices and experiences of individuals from more than twenty countries and from a wide range of networks that one might see as 'European', such as the European AIDS Treatment Group, the International Committee on the Rights of Sex Workers in Europe, and the Eurasian Harm Reduction Association or AIDS Action Europe. Hence, rather than focus exclusively on a single notion of Europe as defined by one particular policy or health-governing entity, the archive's methodology and resulting collected materials reflect a contradictory, dynamic, and unstable notion of Europe as porous, in-the-making, and remarkable in its multiplicity.

Finally, by documenting the narratives of people engaged in the epidemic who have migrated to or from the European region, and the influence of European policies and activities on the states of politics and of the epidemic around the globe, the EHAA is also global in its scale even as its lens is the European region. As such, the concept of Europe that has been mobilised in the archive's initial scope intentionally works to undermine the strengthening of borders and the politics of deserving-ness that characterise that which has come to be called 'Fortress Europe'.[44] Precisely these politics were among the topics at the heart of interviews that we conducted with a variety of interview partners, especially with selected members of the European African Treatment Advocates Network. Archived interviews thereby include multiperspective narrations of migration to and from, as well as within, European countries. These reflect and address the shifting terms of admission and inclusion into legality, health prevention and treatment policies, and citizenship rights and entitlements as generally conceived.

With these three aspects considered together, it becomes clear that labelling and metadata are never purely descriptive. Upon their development and implementation, they immediately introduce analytical dimensions to the ways in which we engage with archived materials. 'What we find is, as ever, contingent on what we set out looking for', wrote the historian Ben Cowan, 'and limited by classificatory systems in which we ourselves are ever more agentive participants'.[45] This reflection is further inspired by Mathias Danbolt's discussion in *Lost and found: queerying the archive* about the necessity to pay attention to the historical discontinuity of concepts and practices, and also to the exclusions that accompany every form of categorisation.[46] The indexing of interviews is therefore not a trivial task, but requires an ongoing discussion about the tensions between today's political claims and historical concepts and contexts.

Conclusion

We regard this sensitivity to the ephemeral, the queer reading, the unhappy archive, and the queering of categorisations as the construction sites necessary to create a queer utopian memory in Muñoz's sense. In *Cruising utopia*, Muñoz sees the political potential of utopias in 'the insistence on potentiality or concrete possibility for another world'.[47] We follow Muñoz in his plea for the essential emotional and political significance of queer utopian memories for today's struggles. We think, however, that the concept of utopia must be complicated by emphasising heterogeneity and dissonances. In addition to empowering and unifying moments of activism, the European HIV/AIDS Archive also documents polyphony, problems, omissions, ignorance, and sometimes the failure of initiatives. It thus allows close readings that unfold the troubling possibilities of thinking that were within reach of contemporary actors, possibilities that the actors skipped over when following the dominant emotional, discursive, and movement practices of their time, when building political coalitions along pre-existing ties and highlighting certain political problems that were near to them but ignoring the realities of other marginalised lives. In this both empowering and critical sense, we believe that the European HIV/AIDS Archive can contribute to what has been termed a *queer counter-memory*.

Acknowledgements

The authors would like to express deep gratitude to all contributors to the EHAA. Thank you for sharing your stories with us. Thank you also to the editors for their helpful feedback on an earlier draft of this chapter. 'Disentangling European HIV/AIDS Policies: Activism, Citizenship and Health' (EUROPACH) is a collaboration between Humboldt-Universität zu Berlin, the University of Basel, Goldsmiths, University of London, and Jagiellonian University, Kraków, and was funded by the Humanities in the European Research Area (HERA.15.093, project duration from 15 September 2016 to 30 November 2019) as part of the joint research programme 'Uses of the Past'. The ' "Don't Criminalize Passion!" The AIDS Crisis and Political Mobilization in the 1980s and early 1990s in Germany' (' "Keine Rechenschaft für Leidenschaft!" Aids-Krise und politische Mobilisierung in den 1980er und frühen 1990er Jahren in Deutschland') (AKPMD) project is funded by the German Research Foundation (Deutsche Forschungsgemeinschaft) (DFG-GZ BI 1353/8–1, project duration from 1 December 2017 to 30 November 2020).

Notes

1 Video interview with Stephen Dressler, conducted in Berlin on 3 July 2018 (in English), available in the European HIV/AIDS Archive, resource ID 118, identifier id_35_ad_ts. This extract comes at the very end of the interview.
2 The archive can be found at: https://rs.cms.hu-berlin.de/ehaa (accessed 8 November 2021).
3 Daniel Marshall, Kevin P. Murphy, and Zeb Tortorici, 'Editors' introduction: queering archives: intimate tracings', *Radical History Review*, 122 (2015), 1–10 (at 9).
4 For example, see the AIDS Collections in the 'Oral history collections at the British Library on the subjects of disability and health' of the British Library (www.bl.uk/collection-guides/oral-histories-of-personal-and-mental-health-and-disability). Additional Europe-based transnational HIV/AIDS archives, although not focused on oral histories, include the collection of AIDS artifacts at the Musée des civilisations de l'europe et de la méditerranée in Marseille (www.mucem.org/page-search?term=sida&type=collection) and the Face of

AIDS Film Archive at the Karolinska Institutet University Library in Stockholm (https://faceofaids.ki.se/about) (all websites accessed 8 November 2021).

5 Steven Epstein, *Impure science: AIDS, activism, and the politics of knowledge* (Berkeley; Los Angeles; London: University of California Press, 1997); Deborah B. Gould, *Moving politics: emotions and ACT UP's fight against AIDS* (Chicago, IL; London: University of Chicago Press, 2009).

6 See, for example, Helen Epstein, *The invisible cure: Africa, the West and the Fight against AIDS* (London: Penguin, 2007); Didier Fassin, *When bodies remember: experiences and politics of AIDS in South Africa* (Berkeley, CA; London: California University Press, 2007); Vinh-Kim Nguyen, 'Antiretroviral globalism, biopolitics, and therapeutic citizenship', in *Global assemblages: technology, politics, and ethics as anthropological problems*, ed. by Aihwa Ong and Stephen J. Collier (Malden, MA: Blackwell Publishing, 2005) pp. 124–44.

7 See, for example, Virginia Berridge, *AIDS in the UK: the making of policy, 1981–1994* (Oxford: Oxford University Press, 1996); Henning Tümmers, *AIDS: Autopsie einer Bedrohung im geteilten Deutschland* (Göttingen: Wallstein Verlag, 2017).

8 For similar considerations regarding an intervention into the dominant narratives of LGBTQI+ history by means of collecting oral histories of diverse populations, see Darnell L. Moore, Beryl Satter, Timothy Stewart-Winter, and Whitney Strub, 'A community's response to the problem of invisibility: the Queer Newark Oral History Project', *QED: A Journal in GLBTQ Worldmaking*, 1.2 (2014), 1–14.

9 Cheryl Ware, '"Things you can't talk about": engaging with HIV-positive gay men's survivor narratives', *Oral History*, 46.2 (2018), 33–40; Wendy Rickard, 'Oral history – "more dangerous than therapy"?: Interviewees' reflections on recording traumatic or taboo issues', *Oral History*, 26.2 (1998), 34–48.

10 Marshall et al., 'Editors' introduction', p. 6.

11 Janet Weston, 'Oral histories, public engagement and the making of positive in prison', *History Workshop Journal*, 87 (2019), 211–23.

12 Available at: www.actuporalhistory.org (accessed 8 November 2021).

13 Emily Jay Nicholls and Marsha Rosengarten carried out the following witness seminars as part of 'Disentangling European HIV/AIDS Policies: Activism, Citizenship and Health' (EUROPACH, 2019): 'Women and HIV in the UK'; 'HIV Prevention and Health Promotion in the UK'; 'The Criminalisation of HIV Transmission in the UK'; 'Antiretroviral Drugs up to and Including Proposition of TasP and PrEP'. Available at: http://europach.phils.uj.edu.pl/project-outcomes/library/witness-seminars/ (accessed 8 November 2021).

14 Zülfukar Çetin and Peter-Paul Bänziger (eds), *Aids und HIV in der Türkei Geschichten und Perspektiven einer emanzipatorischen Gesundheitspolitik* (Gießen: Psychosozial-Verlag, 2019).
15 Information about these exhibitions, including the exhibition catalogue in English, German, Polish, and Turkish, is available on the project's website: europach.phils.uj.edu.pl/project-outcomes/exhibition/ (accessed 8 November 2021).
16 Natalia Ruiz-Junco, 'Feeling social movements: theoretical contributions to social movement research on emotions', *Sociology Compass*, 7.1 (2013), 45–54 (at 52).
17 Beatrice Michaelis, Gabriele Dietze, and Elahe Haschemi Yekani, 'Einleitung: The queerness of things not queer: Entgrenzungen – Affekte und Materialitäten – Interventionen', *Feministische Studien: Zeitschrift für interdisziplinäre Frauen- und Geschlechterforschung*, 30.2 (2012), 184–97 (at 195).
18 José Esteban Muñoz, 'Ghosts of public sex: utopian longings, queer memories', in *Policing public sex: queer politics and the future of AIDS activism*, ed. by Dangerous Bedfellows (Boston, MA: South End Press, 1996), pp. 355–72.
19 José Esteban Muñoz, 'Ephemera as evidence: introductory notes to queer acts', *Women & Performance*, 8.2 (1996), 5–16. See, for example, Ann Cvetkovich, *An archive of feelings: trauma, sexuality, and lesbian public cultures* (Durham, NC: Duke University Press, 2003).
20 Muñoz, 'Ghosts of public sex'.
21 Heather Love, *Feeling backward: loss and the politics of queer history* (Cambridge, MA: Harvard University Press, 2007), p. 32.
22 *Ibid.*
23 Sara Ahmed, 'Killing joy: feminism and the history of happiness', *Signs*, 35.3 (2010), 571–94; Judith Butler, *Precarious life: the powers of mourning and violence* (London; New York: Verso, 2004); Judith Butler, *Frames of war: when life is grievable* (London; New York: Verso, 2009); Jack Halberstam, *The queer art of failure* (Durham, NC: Duke University Press, 2011).
24 Agata Dziuban and Todd Sekuler, 'The temporal regimes of HIV/AIDS activism in Europe: chrono-citizenship, biomedicine and its others', *Critical Public Health*, 31.1 (2021), 5–16.
25 Lauren Berlant, *Cruel optimism* (Durham, NC: Duke University Press, 2011).
26 As cited in Marshall et al., 'Editors' introduction', p. 7.
27 Muñoz, 'Ephemera as evidence'.
28 Mathias Danbolt, 'Touching history: archival relations in queer art and theory', in *Lost and found: queerying the archive*, ed. by Mathias

Danbolt, Jane Rowley, and Louise Wolthers (Copenhagen: Nikolaj, Copenhagen Contemporary Art Center, 2009), pp. 27–45.
29 Muñoz, 'Ephemera as evidence', p. 10. For further reflection on ephemera and archives of HIV/AIDS, see Chapter 9 in this volume.
30 Avery Gordon, *The Hawthorn Archive: letters from the utopian margins* (New York: Fordham University Press, 2018), p. viii.
31 Elizabeth Freeman, *Time binds: queer temporalities, queer histories, perverse modernities* (Durham, NC: Duke University Press, 2010).
32 'Describing an emotion did not always mean feeling it; and conversely an emotion not explicitly articulated might nevertheless be deeply felt', writes Matt Cook with regards to his historical analysis of testimonies of the AIDS crisis in the UK. Matt Cook, ' "Archives of feeling": the AIDS crisis in Britain 1987', *History Workshop Journal*, 83 (2017), 51–78 (at 61).
33 On the psychodynamics between interviewer and interviewee, see Valerie Yow, 'What can oral historians learn from psychotherapists?', *Oral History*, 46.1 (2018), 33–41.
34 Achille Mbembe, *Necropolitics* (Durham, NC: Duke University Press, 2011).
35 Butler, *Frames of war*.
36 Barbara Hobson (ed.), *Recognition struggles and social movements: contested identities, agency and power* (Cambridge: Cambridge University Press, 2003).
37 Donna Haraway, 'Situated knowledges: the science question in feminism and the privilege of partial perspective', *Feminist Studies*, 14.3 (1988), 575–99.
38 Murphy and colleagues use a similar understanding of the term in their discussion of 'what makes queer oral history different', in Kevin P. Murphy, Jennifer L. Pierce, and Jason Ruiz, 'What makes queer oral history different', *The Oral History Review*, 43.1 (2016), 1–24 (at 17).
39 Cathy J. Cohen, 'Punks, bulldaggers, and welfare queens: the radical potential of queer politics?', *GLQ: A Journal of Lesbian and Gay Studies*, 3.4 (1997), 437–65 (at 438).
40 Dipesh Chakrabarty, *Provincialising Europe: postcolonial thought and historical difference* (Princeton, NJ: Princeton University Press, 2000).
41 Joanna Mizielińska and Robert Kulpa, ' "Contemporary peripheries": queer studies, circulation of knowledge and East/West divide', in *De-centring Western sexualities: Central and Eastern European perspectives*, ed. by Robert Kulpa and Joanna Mizielińska (Farnham; Burlington, VT: Ashgate, 2011) pp. 11–26 (at p. 11).

42 Jill Teresa Owczarzak, *Mapping HIV prevention in Poland: contested citizenship and the struggles for health after socialism* (unpublished PhD thesis, University of Kentucky, 2007). Available at: http://uknowledge.uky.edu/gradschool_diss/515 (accessed 8 November 2021).

43 Rasa Navickaité, 'Under the Western gaze: sexuality and postsocialist "transition" in East Europe', in *Postcolonial transitions in Europe: contexts, practices and politics*, ed. by Sandra Ponzanesi and Gianmaria Colpani (London: Rowman & Littlefield, 2016), pp. 119–32 (at p. 128).

44 Nicholas De Genova (ed.), *The borders of "Europe": autonomy of migration, tactics of bordering* (Durham, NC; London: Duke University Press, 2017); Karolina Follis, *Building Fortress Europe: The Polish-Ukrainian border* (Philadelphia: University of Pennsylvania Press, 2012).

45 Ben Cowan, ' "A passive homosexual element": digitized archives and the policing of homosex in Cold War Brazil', *Radical History Review*, 120 (2014), 183–203 (at 198).

46 Danbolt, 'Touching history'.

47 Muñoz, 'Cruising utopia', p. 1.

8

Pandemics and national pride: collecting and curating the history of HIV/AIDS

Manon S. Parry

In 2018, the International AIDS Society (IAS) conference returned to Amsterdam, bringing 18,000 delegates from around the world to a convention centre in the south of the city for lectures, panel discussions, and other activities to disseminate the latest news in research and public health practice.[1] To accompany the event, Amsterdam City Council and the Public Health Service funded a programme of cultural activities for the general public, highlighting the range of AIDS-related work that had been undertaken since the emergence of the pandemic. As an historian of medicine and former museum curator with a long-standing interest in the topic, I undertook several projects to explore the public history of HIV/AIDS, including a pop-up exhibition at the IAS conference, a short film about the early years of the crisis in the Netherlands and living with HIV today, and an international workshop on museum collections, co-hosted with curator Annemarie de Wildt at the Amsterdam Museum.[2]

A recurring theme, at the IAS conference and across the associated activities, was the complexity of addressing the diverse experiences of global HIV/AIDS. In this chapter I focus specifically on the role of museums in this work, and the factors that shape the histories they present. I draw first on the museum workshop, to consider how country contexts shape the collections of objects that have been preserved, and to illustrate some of the common problems encountered across a range of European institutions. I then turn to an exhibition created by the Amsterdam City Archives and displayed there throughout the conference, to demonstrate how public histories of HIV/AIDS tend to privilege certain narratives and exclude other perspectives.[3] Although the exhibition drew on archival materials rather than a museum collection, it exemplifies some of the issues common to both kinds of projects (and indeed most museum exhibitions draw heavily on archival sources and scholarly histories based upon them to shape their particular narratives). To conclude, I reflect on the potential lessons of all of this for the collection and curation of the Covid-19 pandemic.

Archives and museums play a significant role in the formation of cultural memories of HIV/AIDS, with implications for managing the ongoing pandemic as well as for emerging public health challenges. I argue that museums struggle to collect and interpret HIV/AIDS due to the borders and boundaries of their institutional missions, accession policies, and intended audiences. As a result, they create histories that inadequately reflect the diversity of communities and experiences *within* a country, as well as the interactions with other nations that are fundamental characteristics of global pandemics. Such narratives contribute to a widespread underappreciation of the shared risks and responsibilities of contemporary global health.

The history of HIV/AIDS exhibitions in Western Europe and the United States of America (USA) echoes the trajectory of the pandemic since the 1980s, reflecting the ebb and flow of interest in the topic in the Global North once the initial threat was abated by the development of effective drug treatments. Museum exhibitions were part of the activist response from the very beginning, challenging a culture of silence, stigma, and discrimination against people living with HIV/AIDS.[4] For another fifteen years the pandemic continued to generate a wealth of responses as well as collections and exhibitions to document them. Such activities, at least in mainstream venues, decreased dramatically after anti-retroviral medication became available in 1996, creating a 'Second Silence' in the words of curator and critic Theodore Kerr, which lasted well into the first decade of the twentieth century.[5]

During this quieter period, mainstream venues moved on to other topics, although they may have addressed the subject briefly on 1 December annually to mark World AIDS Day, displaying relevant items from their collections or at least blogging about them. This day of commemoration is usually marked by numerous temporary exhibitions showcasing portraits and personal stories of people living with HIV/AIDS, displayed in public venues such as metro systems, town hall buildings, or city streets. In Western Europe, while they may feature some local stories of people from the area, the Global South is commonly depicted as the target area for the most urgent efforts to control HIV/AIDS today.[6]

Historical retrospectives have entrenched this geographical framing. Beginning around 2008, a wave of new projects began, which Kerr and collaborator Alexandra Juhasz have termed 'AIDS Crisis Revisitation', which tended to emphasise the horrors of the early years of the pandemic while celebrating the achievements of AIDS activists, and the impact of scientific breakthroughs.[7] An emphasis on major milestones since the first cases were identified, combined with a narrow focus on the role of gay white men in fighting for HIV/AIDS services, has overshadowed the ongoing impact of the disease as it continues to spread through marginalised communities (even in places where HIV-prevention education is well established and pre-exposure prophylaxis, PrEP, to stop the spread of infection is available). The slogan 'AIDS is not over', widely adopted by AIDS activists and promoted as a core message of the International AIDS Society meeting in Amsterdam in 2018, addresses this tendency to assume that the pandemic is under control – in Western Europe, at least – while the crisis continues elsewhere. Covid-19 has brought renewed attention to the unfinished pandemic caused by HIV/AIDS, although primarily by demonstrating how much we have already forgotten. As I discuss here, European museums are implicated in this process of forgetting despite decades of public histories of HIV/AIDS.

Collecting AIDS

The Amsterdam workshop 'RE:COLLECTIONS – AIDS Objects in Archives and Museums' was intended to take stock of some of the surviving material culture of the history of HIV/AIDS and sketch an outline of the general characteristics of existing collections, drawing on the country-specific knowledge of attending curators, activists, and public historians. Held at the Amsterdam Museum on 26 July 2018, the workshop included twenty-one participants from Belgium, France, Germany, the Netherlands, the United Kingdom

(UK), and the USA. Recognising that all the collections would have particular strengths and weaknesses, participants hoped to identify priorities for future research and ideas for objects which might still be collected. While these conversations only scratched the surface of the public history of HIV/AIDS in each country, they crystallised some of the enduring issues in preserving and interpreting the material culture of the pandemic.

Museums face particular challenges which sharply limit the histories they can preserve and present. This has led to a preponderance of three main types of artefact in museum holdings: artistic, such as a portrait of someone living with HIV/AIDS; activist, such as banners or costumes used in protests; or public-health-related, such as educational posters or pamphlets. These represent only part of the activities undertaken in each realm and reflect only some of the communities affected. Most obviously, and with particular relevance for this book, all attendees acknowledged a lack of diversity in museum collections and in the public histories drawing upon them. The main contributing factors stem from the 'uncontainability' of HIV/AIDS. I focus here on three aspects of this problem: an institution's interpretive mission, its acquisition policies and processes, and its relationship to its specific audiences.

Museum mission

To avoid duplicating efforts elsewhere and to maintain their relevance for their target audiences, all museums establish boundaries regarding what they will collect. While many will have inherited items that are not strictly within this remit (due to a founder's peculiar mix of interests, perhaps, or to save at-risk objects of historical significance until a more suitable home can be found for them), lack of space and resources means that a careful process is needed to weed out multiple versions of the same item, to redistribute collection outliers to other institutions, and to evaluate the importance of potential new acquisitions. While the boundaries used to make such determinations are necessary and logical, they shape museum holdings in sometimes unanticipated ways.

Local history museums, for example, focus on objects and stories with a particular significance for the area around them, or on the local impact of a national or global event. National museums represent a different vantage point, traditionally focusing on people or practices from around the country that are of nationwide significance. A former emphasis on elite figures, especially men in government or military leadership or those known for achievements in the arts or sciences, has broadened in recent years to include everyday stories of a more diverse array of individuals. In medical museums, traditional histories of medical men and their breakthrough discoveries are increasingly told with reference to the contributions of others involved, such as unacknowledged researchers including women who were excluded from professional training or recognition, patients whose lives were affected by a particular illness or experimental treatment, and a wider range of caregivers involved in healthcare. Some are even beginning to incorporate alternative approaches to health and wellbeing, including religious and spiritual healing traditions and complementary medicine, although this remains controversial among some scientists.[8]

Regarding the history of HIV/AIDS, collections typically reflect the character of the epidemic in that country. In contrast to the USA and the UK, for example, where government homophobia restricted the official response to the emerging epidemics there, the Netherlands saw an early coalition between elite gay leaders, public health officials, and the government. A consensus model of decision-making suppressed mass stigmatisation as well as radical activism.[9] As a result, the highly collectible artefacts of public protests were not a major feature of the HIV/AIDS response in the Netherlands. While such items are now preserved in huge collections elsewhere (such as the ACT UP materials at the Museum of European and Mediterranean Civilizations (MuCEM) in Marseille, France, for example), the traces of activism that have survived in Dutch collections are much more limited and are predominantly related to HIV/AIDS prevention education initiatives.[10]

Just as in other countries, health education resources produced by the government as well as grassroots groups are a core component of surviving materials, thanks to mass production and relatively easy storage. There are a number of international poster collections documenting a broad range of approaches from around the world, including more than 10,000 examples now owned by the German Museum of Hygiene in Dresden.[11] Although exhibitions of such examples are common, they rarely document the impact of any particular campaign among those who remember them.[12]

As the Dutch epidemic did not generate a major collecting initiative, historically significant material also appears to have been lost. Examples of valuable artefacts that cannot be located include a scrapbook of photographs and messages from patients, staff, and visitors on one of the first AIDS wards in the country, as well as a handwritten guide to caring for someone with AIDS which was produced by a group looking after their friend and then typed up and distributed in the Dutch buddy system of carers. Personal artefacts that have been saved are mostly associated with well-known people, such as the costumes worn by Hellun Zelluf, a character performed by singer and AIDS activist Geert Vissers (1960–92) as host of *The Gay Dating Show*, a popular television programme which included AIDS-related information.[13] The Dutch version of the AIDS Memorial Quilt includes a more diverse group of people who died of AIDS, and has been split among several museums.[14]

Acquisition policy

Inspired by the NAMES project to commemorate people who have died of AIDS, quilt projects were undertaken in at least thirty-five countries.[15] Although none are as large as the American original, all pose similar challenges for preservation and display. These include the conservation resources required to care for textiles with many different types of items sewn or glued on to the panels; the space and facilities needed to store multiple panels in optimum conditions; the availability of suitable exhibition space to display such large items safely given their high sensitivity to light and the manner in which the materials must be mounted to ensure they are not damaged while on show; and the requirement by most donating groups that panels be made available for reuse in community activities, such as memorial or educational events. The quilts also strain traditional boundaries for collections in terms of categorisation, mixing memorial and activism with art and community history.[16]

HIV/AIDS straddles the boundaries of accessions policies in some settings while failing the admissions criteria of others. For example, at the time of our Amsterdam workshop, the Rijksmuseum

Boerhaave – a museum dedicated to the history of science and medicine – did not include a single item related to HIV/AIDS. A witness seminar organised in June 2014 had failed to generate any objects that would meet the museum's criteria as 'scientific innovations'. As the participants noted, many of the medical breakthroughs came from the application of already-known techniques and technologies for the treatment of HIV/AIDS patients, while other important shifts in healthcare were social rather than medical.[17] The museum is gradually expanding its collection policy to allow for more flexibility in this regard, and as a result has since accessioned a piece of the Dutch AIDS quilt.[18]

Art has been used effectively to bridge the gap in collections which lack personal perspectives and, as collections manager Emma Duggan noted at the 2018 workshop, the Science Museum in London has commissioned new work from artists on a range of topics including AIDS. Even so, acknowledged curator Katie Dabin, of approximately 400 objects in its collection related to HIV/AIDS, around 90 per cent are public health materials. Examples included the same poster and pamphlet materials that dominate in many museum and archive holdings, as well as diagnostic kits for screening blood transfusions that she had collected as part of a wider acquisition of self-test materials in general, and a syringe-dispensing machine developed by a Manchester day centre for drug users.

In our discussion at the workshop, the group noted that a syringe dispenser would have been an ideal item for Dutch collections given that the Netherlands was the first country in the world to institute a needle exchange programme as a means to slow the spread of HIV/AIDS among intravenous drug users. Yet such an item has not been collected, and in fact Dutch attendees could not recall if they were used during the most urgent era of the epidemic. We even considered the prospect that they might not have been needed, assuming that Dutch investment in the public health response would have been greater than in the UK and so personnel may have been paid to distribute syringes instead. As images in the Amsterdam City Archive later revealed, dispensing machines were indeed used in the city, yet the lack of familiarity with this among Dutch workshop attendees reveals just how quickly history can disappear from memory. Our discussion was also significant in revealing how notions of national cultures and values can fuel misleading assumptions about the past.

An important outcome of the 2018 workshop was the donation of a piece of the Dutch AIDS quilt to the London Science Museum, as an example of the wider global impact of the pandemic as well as the links between London and Amsterdam's gay scenes and the relationships that emerged between people travelling between the two cities.[19]

Another major gap in collections relates to medical initiatives that did not succeed, as well as fake cures marketed commercially. Useless or dangerous products advertised as preventative or curative represent an important part of the history of responses to HIV/AIDS, but fall outside the scope of museums focused on scientifically proven treatments. Yet such artifacts offer opportunities to address the historical myths as well as the market for misinformation that continues today. Gerard Koskovich, of the GLBT Historical Society Museum and Archives in San Francisco, noted, for example, that the selection of poppers housed in their collection could be used to address stigma and myths about 'gay lifestyle' as well as early theories about the role of drug use as a possible contributor to AIDS-related illnesses, as well as HIV/AIDS denialism.[20]

Women's histories of HIV/AIDS are severely underrepresented in existing collections in general, reflecting the wider lack of attention to women's history in museums, and women's health in particular. As workshop attendees from the International Community of Women Living with HIV/AIDS pointed out, microbicide research is a 'forgotten history' within the common narratives of the development of medical interventions for HIV/AIDS. In fact, the tendency to highlight progress leaves unsuccessful or unpopular research out of the timeline of scientific research and discovery entirely.[21]

Museum audiences

Collecting the history of HIV/AIDS among drug users and other marginalised groups such as sex workers has proven particularly difficult for most museums, meaning that their perspectives are very rarely part of public exhibitions. Florent Molle and Renaud Chantraine of MuCEM reported that white gay men are best represented in the holdings of 12,000 HIV/AIDS-related objects gathered between 2002 and 2006, just as elsewhere. ACT UP played a dominant role in challenging government inaction and remains dominant in the prevailing historical memory of the epidemic there.[22]

The limitations of HIV/AIDS protest collections elsewhere are coming into view, however, amid discussion among curators about the limited range of activism that is visible, collectible, and exhibitable. A focus on the witty signs, colourful props, spectacular acts, and media records of direct action has obscured the wider role of activities required to generate and maintain major shifts in policy and funding. In this way, the contributions of people who are not part of the most media- (and museum-) friendly front stage of the action but who are equally invested and influential behind the scenes are ignored. This theme was taken up in a subsequent workshop organised at the Science Museum in London in 2019, on 'The Material Culture of Health Care Activism', where several speakers emphasised the need to expand definitions of what 'counts' as activism, alongside the importance of 'contemporary collecting' in the midst of a controversy or crisis in order to capture material that might be otherwise lost or destroyed.[23]

In an attempt to enrich existing collections, some archives and museums are taking up retrospective projects to encourage new donations and record oral histories from previously excluded communities. 'Community-curated' projects invite underrepresented groups to participate in the creation of new exhibitions, although the degree of real collaboration is highly variable and such projects have been criticised for a range of pitfalls, from limiting the degree of actual participation or using collaborators to deflect criticism, to presenting only favourable or simplistic histories dominated by community leaders without acknowledging a more diverse range of perspectives within the wider group.[24] Although few museums use an explicitly 'iterative' approach to exhibitions by inviting represented groups to critique and revise displays after their initial launch, new accessions may well be identified and donated as a result of someone's dissatisfaction with a finished project. Curators also commonly use exhibitions as a way to address gaps in the collection and to reach out to underrepresented groups to build relationships and try to identify relevant artefacts for preservation.

MuCEM has held a series of community consultations to try and broaden the range of perspectives they can include, yet the most vulnerable groups (such as drug users and recent migrants) have not participated, largely due to a lack of enthusiasm for working 'within' the institution. In the USA, I encountered similar hesitancy among activists when researching a National Library of Medicine exhibition, with many reluctant to tell their stories or lend their materials to a government institution. During research for the 2018 film project on HIV/AIDS in the Netherlands, our team also noted a great deal of nervousness among people living with HIV or using PrEP about being identifiable on film, revealing ongoing stigma belied by cultural narratives of 'Dutch tolerance' and the celebratory storylines common in histories of progress in the HIV/AIDS pandemic. The predominantly white, middle-class profile of museum employees is increasingly cited as a factor in the lack of diverse perspectives represented in museum collections and exhibitions.[25] Such homogeneity makes it difficult for many institutions to build credible collaborations with a range of partners. Projects attempting to 'share authority' with communities outside of the museum are often disappointing for all involved, given the difficulties of integrating different expectations, practices, and priorities, especially in the context of tight deadlines and limited budgets.[26]

A final challenge, raised by Gerard Koskovich, is the role of grief and remembrance in limiting museum collections. One of the reasons it has been difficult to collect personal items that represent lived experiences is that people hold on to objects that remind them of loved ones who have died. In San Francisco, friends were commonly welcomed into a person's apartment after their death and invited to take items, partly in remembrance and to ease the burden of a surviving partner, but also to dispose of the belongings of individuals (who may have been estranged from their families). When the people now treasuring these objects also die, their origins and historical significance may not be known to their heirs and descendants, further decreasing the likelihood that they will be donated to museums or saved with contextualising documentation.[27]

As I have shown here, public histories are heavily circumscribed by the mission of their host institution, the collections contained therein, and the audiences they attract. In the next section I turn to a specific example, to consider some of the consequences of collecting habits for the interpretation of the history of HIV/AIDS in an exhibition.

Pandemics and national pride 225

Exhibiting AIDS

AIDS in Amsterdam, 1981–1996 was displayed at the Amsterdam City Archives from 6 July to 2 September 2018, during the IAS conference, and was open to the general public as well as conference-goers. The exhibition consisted of a series of panels of reproductions of images and documents from the archives and a row of pieces of the Dutch AIDS quilt displayed above them, hanging from the ceiling. The panels were titled thematically and the narrative followed a chronology, from the first patient with an unknown illness in 1981 to the introduction of combination therapy in 1996. Along the bottom of the exhibition structure, the rising number of deaths from AIDS in the Netherlands was listed, corresponding with the timeline in the panels.

The exhibition text focused explicitly on Amsterdam as the core of the Dutch experience of the pandemic and emphasised throughout the famously 'progressive' approach of the Netherlands and the leading role of gay rights organisations in the response. Most of the country's cases occurred in the city, which was the centre of gay life nationally as well as a popular international destination. As the introduction to the exhibition also noted, 'several sections of the population were at increased risk of infection', which is explained in a subsequent panel reporting that around 10,000 heroin users and 5,000–6,000 active sex workers lived in the city in the 1980s.

The first panel included headlines asserting the greatest impact of HIV/AIDS in Amsterdam, accompanied by a large image of a public health poster 'specifically targeting tourists and visitors'. The poster, shown in Figure 8.1, features a black-and-white photograph of two men involved in a sexual encounter with the familiar buildings of the old centre of the city clearly visible in the background. In the foreground, one man lies naked on his stomach on a bed while the other, wearing only his underwear, looks down at him. A red banner of text reads 'Amsterdam is yours' followed by the words 'keep it safe'. The accompanying caption noted that the poster was produced by a collaboration between 'the management of Amsterdam's gay bars and discos and Amsterdam's Gay AIDS information group', underlining the joint role of officials and at-risk communities in the Dutch response. The prominence of the naked man's body in the centre of the image represents a clear contrast

226 Histories of HIV/AIDS in Western Europe

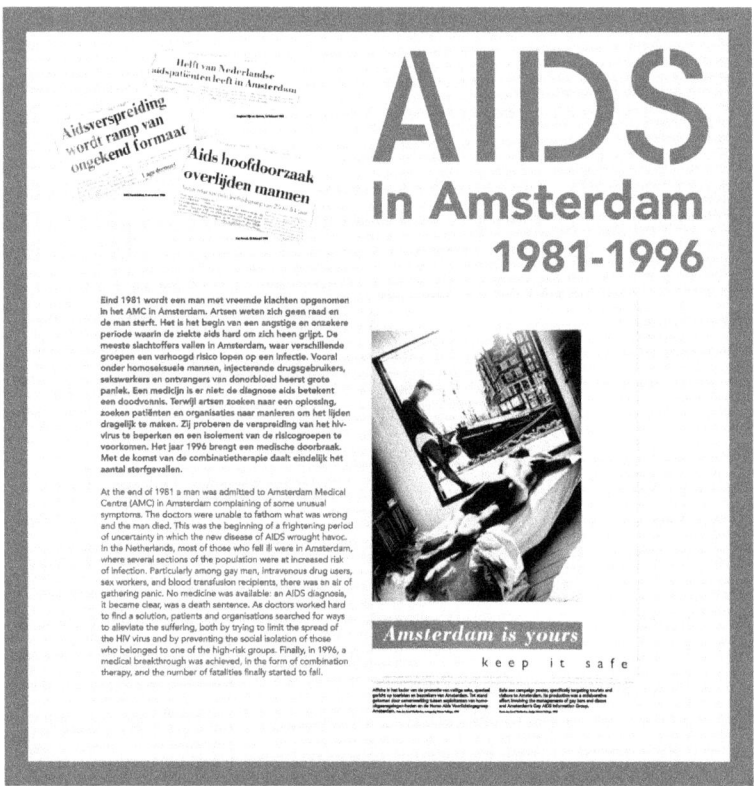

Figure 8.1 First panel of the exhibition *AIDS in Amsterdam, 1981–1996*, Amsterdam City Archives, 2018. Courtesy of exhibition designer Jasper van Goor and Amsterdam City Archives.

with the silences and euphemisms common in other countries' HIV/AIDS prevention campaigns. Such candour is presumably thanks to the collaborative public health strategy combined with the celebrated 'tolerance' commonly attributed to Dutch society.

The exhibition's introductory text characterised 1981 as 'the beginning of a frightening period of uncertainty in which the new disease of AIDS wrought havoc'. It went on to describe the years before effective treatment, rising panic, the efforts of doctors 'to find a solution', and the work of patients and organisations to 'alleviate suffering' by preventing the spread of the virus as well as

Pandemics and national pride 227

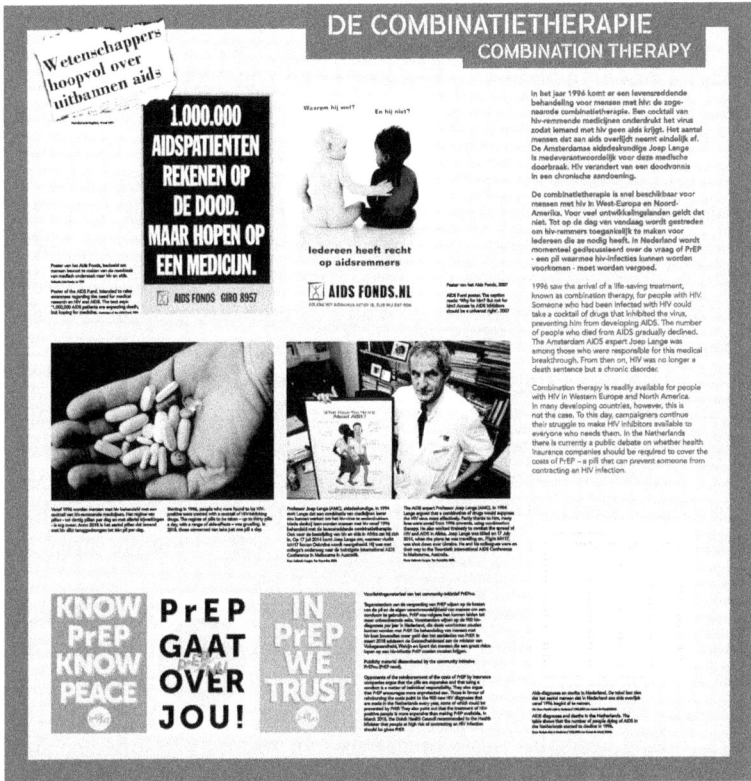

Figure 8.2 Last panel of the exhibition *AIDS in Amsterdam, 1981–1996*, Amsterdam City Archives, 2018. Courtesy of exhibition designer Jasper van Goor and Amsterdam City Archives.

addressing the social isolation of those most at risk. This first panel ended with a positive outcome, saying, '[f]inally, in 1996, a medical breakthrough was achieved, in the form of combination therapy, and the number of fatalities finally started to fall'.

The final panel of the exhibition, shown in Figure 8.2, presented a more inconclusive message, however. Under the heading 'Combination Therapy', this section described its development, featuring 'Amsterdam AIDS expert Joep Lange [who] was among those who were responsible for this medical breakthrough'. The text noted that while the treatment 'is readily available for people with HIV in Western Europe and North America ... [i]n many developing countries, however, this is not the case'. The other images shown include a 2007 poster from Dutch charitable organisation AIDS Fonds depicting a white and a Black toddler sitting together, shown from behind, with the white child's hand gently reaching around the back of his companion. Above the two, in Dutch, the text asks, 'Why him? And not him?', followed by the statement that everyone has the right to AIDS inhibitors, referencing unequal global access to HIV/AIDS drugs and visually reinforcing the idea that the (white) Dutch are responsible for 'helping' the Black 'other'. The concluding images include publicity materials promoting the use of pre-exposure prophylaxis, accompanied by an explanation of the Dutch debate over insurance companies' responsibility to reimburse policyholders who use these drugs to prevent infection with HIV. The section concluded with the March 2018 recommendation to the government that PrEP should be provided free to those at risk, although this was not actually taken up.[28]

Several places in the exhibition drew specific attention to Dutch individuals or activities as particularly important milestones in the history of the pandemic. The first section, 'Gay Capital', so titled to emphasise the importance of the city in global gay culture, highlighted the work of activists in promoting safe sex and raising money for research and services for people with HIV/AIDS. The next section, 'Condoms and Clean Needles', focused on the country's introduction of the world's first needle exchange programme in 1984, although a later section implies this was not universal as it includes protests to make clean needles available to prisoners in 1991. This section also mentioned the 'tolerant attitude to street prostitution', including HIV/AIDS education campaigns for sex workers, as well as a hint of the limits of this tolerance in a reference to city residents' protests highlighting the negative impact of prostitution in their communities. As shown elsewhere in this book, both prisons and sex work tested the limits of tolerant, liberal, or collaborative responses to HIV/AIDS.

The section on action groups featured protests at the American consulate over restrictions on immigration for people with HIV/AIDS, and the 1992 IAS conference in Amsterdam – which was relocated to the Netherlands in response to US travel rules restricting entry for people with HIV/AIDS. Although this was not explicitly mentioned in the text, it was likely to have been very well known among conference attendees, who were encouraged to visit the exhibition. The panel text concluded that 'The Netherlands was widely praised for its AIDS policy.' Joep Lange is mentioned three times, celebrated for his research and for working 'tirelessly to combat the spread of HIV/AIDS in Africa'. The concluding panel also noted that he was killed on 17 July 2014, 'when the plane he was traveling on, MH17, was shot down over Ukraine'. Many passengers on this flight were HIV/AIDS researchers or activists heading to the twentieth IAS conference in Melbourne, Australia, so the inclusion of this detail likely resonated with visiting attendees, as well as with Dutch audiences who participated in national memorial activities to commemorate the 193 Dutch victims (more than two-thirds of those on board).

The largest section of the exhibition, 'From HIV to AIDS', occupied three panels, where most were on two. They featured photographs of people at parties and events for those living with AIDS, and images of people with advanced disease at home or in care facilities – with most identified by name. Subsequent sections on 'New Funeral Culture' and 'Commemoration' similarly highlighted the impact of the Dutch epidemic by including the names of people who had died or who had participated in various memorial activities.

Links to the global pandemic are made in this section through references to the 'AIDS Memorial Quilt' which inspired the Dutch version displayed with the exhibition; tourism; '[t]he new disease that arrived from the United States'; and the global inequality in access to HIV/AIDS drugs. Overwhelmingly, though, the narrative focuses on the Netherlands, and within that primarily on white gay men. The origins of the disease are located elsewhere (in the USA) and the role of visitors in spreading the infection is also emphasised. The main impression is that the crisis is over, and the concluding panel suggests the main challenge now lies elsewhere – in Africa – where the Dutch can also play a role.

Many of these elements reflect the scope dictated by the source material, the location of the exhibition, and the occasion for its display, being the return of the IAS conference to Amsterdam. Yet the narrative also follows the conventions of most public histories of HIV/AIDS at other museums across Western Europe and the USA, by including a timeline (which highlights a rising death toll as well as scientific developments) and focusing primarily on technical solutions, with less attention to the structural issues that place some at more risk of infection than others. Some home communities are overlooked – as they are elsewhere – including women with HIV/AIDS and people with haemophilia. By ending the story in 1996 and concluding with the challenge of HIV/AIDS in Africa, the exhibition also ignores the ongoing challenge of new infections in the Netherlands and the return of stigma.

Conclusion: Covid-19 and the resurgence of national narratives

Since HIV infection shifted from a life-threatening issue to a chronic condition in Western Europe, the topic has held a declining place in priorities for collecting and exhibiting the history of pandemics. HIV/AIDS is hardly present in the public health section of the London Science Museum's newly renovated Medicine Galleries, the world's largest history-of-medicine exhibition, showcasing more than 3,000 objects in over 3,000 square metres.[29] The hundredth anniversary of the 1918 influenza pandemic in 2018 saw a wave of new exhibitions on the risks of (re-)emerging infectious diseases, where HIV/AIDS competed for audience attention amidst Ebola, SARS, and the looming threat of a new pandemic. A year later the new pandemic emerged with the global spread of Covid-19. As historians and AIDS activists have noted, the response suggests that few of the most important lessons of the history of HIV/AIDS have actually been learnt, and some have forgotten completely about the 'unfinished' pandemic of HIV.[30]

Despite the shared threat across borders and the collaborative effort needed to contain the spread, nationalistic discourses have dominated. Amidst many countries' responses of closing borders and blaming foreigners, the Dutch government insisted that the country's 'sober' culture allowed them to implement a more 'intelligent lockdown' than in other regions.[31] Yet European populations are diverse *within* as well as *across* country borders. Public histories can play a role in broadening such narrow perspectives, but only if relevant collections of material culture, and the individual stories associated with them, have survived. Museums need to consider how to better capture the global dimensions even when focusing on their immediate target community, and any exhibition beginning from the relevance for local communities might overstate supposedly unique elements while overlooking the international connections.

HIV/AIDS powerfully demonstrated the interlocking social, economic, political, cultural, and historical factors that shape individual risk as well as the global management of infectious-disease pandemics. Covid-19 requires a similarly complex view. A focus only on the medical issues, highlighting the structure of the virus, the ways infections spreads, and the timeline of 'discoveries' made would obscure aspects of the early months that help to explain other important dimensions, such as why some communities were harder hit, how contradictory information muddied health advice and fuelled non-compliance, and how scientific conflict and cooperation played out across countries. A social history emphasising the range of community responses, such as banners supporting essential workers and pictures hung in windows to encourage positivity, might capture the most well-publicised activities, but misses less media-friendly efforts, those on a smaller scale, and more distressing experiences of isolation and loss.

A plethora of online platforms have been launched to capture the impact of Covid-19 across different groups. The surge in digital communication fuelled by bans on travel, the closure of workplaces and educational institutions, and the call for people to stay home have made such digital collecting a priority now that so much of life is lived online, as well as a necessity given the restrictions on movement and meeting up. The scale of stories that can be captured in this manner is impressive, and there is an array of projects targeting specific groups such as students, healthcare workers, and people with disabilities. However, unless this approach is supplemented by additional activities to collect objects, silences in the public histories will persist, especially for groups without easy access to digital tools, including older people as well as poorer people and those living in institutional settings such as care homes, prisons, and mental health facilities. This is an especially important issue given that all of these groups face particular risks in this pandemic.

While we could mine digital collections for ideas for objects to be accessioned by museums, some may disappear before curators can reach individuals, if they can contact them at all, to ask that such items be saved for the future.

Although museum staff are discussing collecting strategies, a heavy emphasis has been placed on 'ethical approaches' so as not to distract essential workers in healthcare especially from their core priorities, or to burden those dealing with grief with museum priorities. Yet, in the midst of a crisis, materials that are no longer medically useful may be discarded, and more personal items may be dismissed as insignificant rather than valuable for the historical record. A key strategy that is needed, then, is the cultivation of 'historical consciousness' to encourage people across different communities to see themselves as part of history in the making, and to reach out to those groups likely to be underrepresented with other kinds of collecting initiatives. If we assume that the scale of the crisis is large enough to ensure its preservation in the historical record, and neglect the need to gather a broad range of materials to reflect the diversity of its impact, the end result, as with HIV/AIDS, may be a narrow picture of the past with limited relevance for preparing for the future.

Notes

1 International AIDS Society, 'AIDS 2018', available online at: www.aids2018.org (accessed 11 March 2022); see also amsterdam&partners, *Jaarverslaag 2018* (Amsterdam: amsterdam&partners, 2018), p. 27, available online at: https://issuu.com/iamsterdam/docs/jaarverslag_amsterdam_partners_2018 (accessed 11 March 2022).

2 *Voices of the Epidemic* (film, 2018), available online at: www.manonparry.com/films/voices-of-the-epidemic-2018 (accessed 11 March 2022); *Rights and Responsibilities: AIDS in the Netherlands*, pop-up exhibition displayed at the International AIDS Society Conference, Amsterdam, July 2018.

3 *Aids in Amsterdam, 1981–1996*, exhibition, 6 July–2 September 2018: www.amsterdam.nl/stadsarchief/agenda/aids (accessed 11 March 2022).

4 Douglas Crimp, 'AIDS: cultural analysis/cultural activism', in *Melancholia and moralism* (Cambridge, MA: The MIT Press, 2002), pp. 27–41. Originally published in *October 43* (Winter 1987), 3–16.

5 Theodore (ted) Kerr, 'What you don't know about AIDS could fill a museum: curatorial ethics and the ongoing epidemic in the 21st century', *On Curating*, 42 (2019), 5–13.
6 National AIDS Trust, 'World AIDS Day', www.worldaidsday.org (accessed 11 March 2022). See, for example, Ben Norum, 'World AIDS Day – positive living: art and AIDS in South Africa exhibition at Birkbeck University', *GO LONDON newsletter*, 1 December 2015, available at www.standard.co.uk/culture/exhibitions/world-aids-day-positive-living-art-and-aids-in-south-africa-exhibition-at-birkbeck-university-a3126851.html (accessed 9 March 2022); United Nations in the Russian Federation, 'Announcement! Photo exhibition "Stars against AIDS" on World AIDS Day', n.d., available at: www.unrussia.ru/en/un-in-russia/news/2008-11-27 (accessed 11 March 2022); Saisha, 'World AIDS Day', Smithsonian American Art Museum, 1 December 2018, https://americanart.si.edu/blog/eye-level/2018/01/58106/world-aids-day (accessed 11 March 2022).
7 Alexandra Juhasz and Theodore Kerr, 'Who are the stewards of the AIDS archive? Sharing the political weight of the intimate', in *The unfinished queer agenda after marriage equality*, ed. by Angela Jones and Joseph Nicholas DeFilippis (New York: Routledge, 2018), pp. 88–101.
8 See, for example, the Science Museum's newly renovated Medicine Galleries which opened in 2019.
9 Gert Hekma and Jan Willem Duyvendak, 'The Netherlands, depoliticization of homosexuality and homosexualisation of politics', in *Queer theory/sociology*, ed. by Steven Seidman (Maiden, MA: Blackwell, 1996), pp. 421–38. See also Chapter 1 in this collection for another example of national policy drawing to a large extent on consensus and collaboration.
10 Renaud Chantraine, Florent Molle, and Sandrine Musso, 'AIDS politics of representation and narratives: a current project at the Museum of European and Mediterranean Civilizations (Mucem) in Marseille, France', *On Curating*, 42 (2019), 206–18.
11 This collection was used as the basis of the recent exhibition *AIDS: Based On A True Story*, displayed there in 2015–16 and at the International Museum of the Red Cross from 2017 to 2018. See Vladimir Ĉajkovac (ed.), *AIDS: based on a true story*, trans. by Stephen Grynwasser (Dresden: Verlag des Deutschen Hygiene-Museums, 2015).
12 Manon S. Parry, 'Public health heritage and policy: HIV and AIDS in museums and archives', *História, Ciências, Saúde-Manguinhos*, 27 (supplement 1) (2020), 253–62.

13 Amsterdam Museum, 'Outfit van Hellun Zelluf, Driedelig', n.d., https://hart.amsterdam/nl/collectie/object/amcollect/99209 (accessed 11 March 2022).
14 Léontine Meijer-van Mensch and Annemarie de Wildt, 'AIDS memorial quilts: from mourning and activism to heritage objects', in *Die Musealisierung der Gegenwart. Von Grenzen und Chancen des Sammelns in Kulturhistorischen Museen*, ed. by Sophie Elpers and Anna Palm (Bielefeld: transcript, 2014) pp. 63–82.
15 Elizabeth Fee, 'The AIDS memorial quilt', *American Journal of Public Health*, 96.6 (2006), 979.
16 Iona Literat and Anne Balsamo, 'Stitching the future of the AIDS quilt: the cultural work of digital memorials', *Visual Communication Quarterly*, 21.3 (2014), 138–49.
17 Manon S. Parry and Hugo Schalkwijk, 'Lost objects and missing histories: HIV/AIDS in the Netherlands', in *Activism, unruliness, and alterity: gender, sexuality and museums*, Vol. 2, ed. by Joshua G. Adair and Amy K. Levin (London; New York: Routledge, 2020), pp. 113–26.
18 Personal communication with curator Mieneke te Hennepe, 2 March 2020.
19 Thanks to a collaboration between Jörn Wolters of the Stichting NAMENproject Nederland, and Katie Dabin and Imogen Clarke.
20 GLBT Historical Society, 'The GLBT Historical Society Museum', www.glbthistory.org/museum-about-visitor-info (accessed 11 March 2022).
21 Patricia Kingori and Salla Sariola, 'Museum of failed HIV research', *Anthropology & Medicine*, 22.3 (2015), 213–16. On women's experiences and activism, see Chapter 6 in this book.
22 Chantraine et al., 'AIDS politics of representation and narratives'.
23 'The Material Culture of Health Activism', workshop held in London on 20 June 2019; see ArtHist.net listing, 18 May 2019: https://arthist.net/archive/20856 (accessed 31 August 2020).
24 Bernadette Lynch, Sarah Smed, Adele Chynoweth, and Klaus Petersen (eds), *Museums and social change: challenging the unhelpful museum* (London; New York: Routledge, 2020).
25 Manuel Charr, 'Museums and employee diversity', *MuseumNext*, 24 August 2019, www.museumnext.com/article/museums-and-employee-diversity/ (accessed 31 August 2020).
26 Bill Adair, Benjamin Filene, and Laura Koloski (eds), *Letting go? Sharing historical authority in a user-generated world* (Philadelphia, PA: Pew Center for Arts and Heritage, 2011).
27 Thanks to Janet Weston for this observation.
28 Instead, in 2019, local councils in the Netherlands began a five-year programme to distribute PrEP.

29 Science Museum, 'World's largest medicine galleries open at the Science Museum', 4 November 2019, www.sciencemuseum.org.uk/about-us/press-office/worlds-largest-medicine-galleries-open-science-museum-0 (accessed 31 August 2020).

30 Guillaume Lachenal and Gaëtan Thomas, 'COVID-19: when history has no lessons', History Workshop Online, 30 March 2020, www.historyworkshop.org.uk/covid-19-when-history-has-no-lessons and Virginia Berridge, 'History does have something to say', History Workshop Online, 20 May 2020, www.historyworkshop.org.uk/history-does-have-something-to-say/ (both accessed 31 August 2020).

31 Reuters Staff, 'Dutch PM Rutte: ban on public gatherings is "intelligent lockdown"', Reuters, 23 March 2020, www.reuters.com/article/us-health-coronavirus-netherlands-gather/dutch-pm-rutte-ban-on-public-gatherings-is-intelligent-lockdown-idUSKBN21A39V (accessed 24 March 2020); Wouter Kempenaar, 'Nederlanders "trots" en "nuchter"? Onzin, zegt Vlaming Tom Lanoye', NPO Radio 1, 5 August 2020, www.nporadio1.nl/gezondheid/25622-in-nederland-is-eer-een-zekere-koppigheid-in-bestrijding-corona (accessed 5 August 2020).

Index

acquired immune deficiency syndrome (AIDS) *see* HIV/AIDS
activism 1–2, 5, 7, 14–19, 125, 169, 186, 194–8, 205–7, 209, 219–20, 223
   collaborative 17–18, 144, 164–7
   gay men's 6, 167
   prison 82, 84, 89, 95, 97–8, 100–1
   sex workers' 28–9, 50
activists 12, 15, 28, 30, 46, 62, 77, 126, 176, 193–4, 196–7, 200–2, 216–18, 224, 228–30
   interviews with 27, 50, 198–9, 202, 206
   LGBT 32, 49, 167
   networks 13, 196
   organisations 121, 180, 182, 186
   patients 122–3
   sex workers 49–50
addiction 10–11, 61, 72, 77, 83–4, 91–4, 97, 99, 115, 177
   services 83, 99
   work 84, 91–4, 101
addicts 11, 31, 65, 119, 171, 177
advertising 3, 47, 69–72, 111, 113, 145, 170
Africa 10–11, 229–30
agency 123, 166, 171
AIDS *see* HIV/AIDS

AIDS Memorial Quilt 220–2, 225, 229
Aiuti, Dr Fernando 62–63, 77
Amsterdam 8–9, 12, 20, 88, 215, 217, 220–2, 225–9
antiretroviral therapy 4, 110
anxiety 1, 11, 16, 33, 46, 86, 113, 116, 129–30, 142, 146, 148–9, 154–5, 177–8
   public 15, 82, 144
   social 73, 153
archive(s) 1–2, 7–8, 15, 19–21, 27, 50, 141, 153, 164–6, 193–4, 196, 200–1, 203, 205, 207, 209, 216, 221, 223
   see also European HIV/AIDS Archive
artefacts 218–20, 223
attitudes 19, 33, 43, 94, 111–12, 115, 139, 144, 155, 173, 208
   changing 4, 95, 122
   public 18, 151–2
authorities 27–8, 31, 33, 43–6, 98
   health 5, 27, 41, 72, 144–6, 150

babies 171–2, 174–6, 178–9, 180–1
   see also childbirth
backlash 6, 46, 130, 201–2
Barnardo's 179, 184
bars 41, 155, 225
Berlin 85, 199

Berne 8, 96–8, 100
biomedicine 1, 4–5, 18, 131, 198
  see also medicine
blood 33, 37, 65, 67, 69, 118, 139, 144–5, 168, 174, 178–9
  donation 32, 67, 119, 144
  transfusion 32, 39, 114, 121, 144, 221
books 183–4
  children's 8, 19, 178, 184
  picture 165, 183–4
boundaries 20, 27, 84, 98, 100, 125, 129, 156, 171, 207, 216, 218, 220
Britain *see* United Kingdom (UK)

callers to helplines 139, 150, 153–5
campaign(s) 1, 3–4, 6, 15, 37, 50, 68, 72, 140, 142, 151, 173, 202, 220, 226
  information 3, 17, 33, 47, 113–14, 142, 145–6, 153, 168–70, 228
Cardiff 140, 142–5, 148, 150–1, 153–5
Caritas 60–3
Casa famiglia 59–67, 71–2
charities 3, 14, 146–7, 150, 170, 173, 179, 184
childbirth 172, 175–7
  see also babies
children 5, 8, 16, 19, 37, 39, 60, 64, 66, 146
  HIV-affected 165–9, 173–4, 176–86
  HIV-infected 170, 172, 174, 179–81, 183, 198
church 17, 60–80, 92, 114
collaboration 17, 19, 28, 49–50, 72, 75, 111, 180, 182, 197, 223–6, 228, 230
  care 121, 123, 125, 131–2, 164
  combination therapy 225, 227
community 48, 60, 67, 82, 85, 90, 93, 97, 99, 100–1, 111, 117, 129, 142, 194, 201–2, 205–6, 216–17, 223–4, 228, 231–2
  action 3, 6, 112, 140, 142–3, 151, 220
  affected 5, 20, 46, 50, 127, 193, 205, 218, 225, 230–1
  global 15, 74
  LGBT 49, 110, 117–19, 202
  services 6, 93, 95, 99, 100, 117, 142, 147, 157, 176
compassion 118, 120, 132
condoms 48, 68–9, 97–8, 156, 202
  in prison 83–5, 89–91, 104
  in sex work 39–42, 44–6, 49
confidentiality 13, 100, 115, 145, 152, 182, 185
  medical 83, 93, 97, 127
conversation 61, 74, 94
  between parents and children 165, 184–5
  difficult 184–5
Cook, Matt 113, 130, 153
Council of Europe 83–5, 93, 100
Covid-19 77, 216–17, 230–1
Craxi, Bettino 59, 73–7
crime 9
  hate 119
  organised 74–5, 77
criminalisation 13, 198, 201
  drugs 73, 75–7
  HIV/AIDS 4, 60, 98
  sex education 202
  sex work 28–9, 50
Cutting, Dr William 179–80, 182
  see also Paediatric AIDS Resource Centre

death 34, 74, 93, 110, 113, 119–20, 130, 153, 171, 173, 185, 198, 205, 224
  machine 34, 36–7
  penalty 73, 76
  rate 1, 4, 116, 193, 225, 230
Directorate of Health (Norway) 33, 43, 45–8
dirty work 110, 124
disinfectant 85, 90, 95, 99, 149

doctors 27, 30, 89, 92–3, 140, 172, 174, 179–82, 226
   Italian 62, 66, 68, 72
   prison 17, 97, 99–100
Donat-Cattin, Carlo 67–9, 71–2
drug(s) 6, 10, 31, 65, 91, 147, 195, 198
   dealers 65–6, 73–4, 76
   legislation 59, 73, 76–7
   policy 6, 11, 17, 42, 74–6, 194
   in prison 17, 82, 83–5, 90–5, 99
   treatment 83, 94
   use 13, 29–31, 34, 61, 72–4, 76–7, 96–8, 121, 152, 169, 182, 198, 222
   users 2–3, 6, 11–12, 15–17, 19–20, 31, 33, 40–4, 59–61, 65–7, 69, 71–2, 77, 95, 101, 120, 125, 128, 168, 170–2, 176–7, 194, 198, 205, 221–2, 224
   war on 17, 59, 73–5, 77
   see also addiction; addicts
Dublin 17, 87, 92, 94, 96, 99

EATG *see* European AIDS Treatment Group (EATG)
ECS *see* European Collaborative Study (ECS)
Edinburgh 2, 8, 9, 11–13, 19, 120, 128, 140, 146, 164–79, 182, 185–6
education 16, 42, 65, 82, 84–5, 88–9, 91, 94, 100, 146–7, 149, 156, 170–1, 174, 179, 182–3, 186, 220
   health 13, 18, 30, 139, 142, 167–9, 217, 219, 228
   materials 44, 145, 147, 174, 218
   peer 17, 45
   sex 45, 143, 147, 156, 202
EHAA *see* European HIV/AIDS Archive (EHAA)
emotion(s) 14, 30, 115–16, 129–32, 141, 153–5, 166–7, 174–5, 184–5, 197, 204, 209

emotional labour 119
emotional needs 19, 165, 170, 178–9, 186
England 18, 86–7, 89–90, 150, 167, 169
   see also United Kingdom (UK)
environment
   care 121–2, 125–6, 131
   home-like 110, 126
ephemera 1, 8, 153, 193, 203, 205, 209
epidemic, HIV/AIDS 1–2, 4, 10, 14, 17–18, 31–4, 37, 39, 42–3, 46, 49–50, 61–2, 72, 77, 91–2, 96, 153, 195–6, 200, 207, 219–21
   development of 15, 28, 32, 155–6, 168, 171–2, 194, 205
   histories of 8, 14, 82, 193–4, 223
   impact of 12, 27, 33, 50, 84, 120, 172, 193, 229
   narratives of 5, 39, 59, 171, 193, 205, 208
   see also pandemic, HIV/AIDS
EPSP *see* European Peer Support Project (EPSP)
EUROPACH 196, 199, 204, 210
European AIDS Treatment Group (EATG) 193–4, 208
European Collaborative Study (ECS) 176, 179
European HIV/AIDS Archive (EHAA) 19–20, 192–210
European Peer Support Project (EPSP) 94–5, 99
exhibitions 1, 7–8, 20, 199, 215–16, 219–20, 222–31
experience(s) 2, 5, 7, 15–19, 21, 43, 45, 94–5, 101, 110–12, 118–23, 126, 130–1, 139–40, 143, 151–2, 157, 164–5, 168–70, 172–3, 182, 185–6, 192–3, 198, 201–2, 204–6
   birth 175, 177
   difficult 40, 116, 231

Index

diversity of 12–13, 22, 94, 140, 195, 200, 206, 208, 215–16
expertise by 14–15, 111, 121–2
lived 121, 166–7, 194, 196–7, 206, 224
non-normative 203, 205
expertise 6, 15, 83, 167, 169, 173–4, 182
  by experience 14–15, 111, 121–2
  medical 99, 185–6
  patient 6, 18

families 19, 39, 59–61, 64–5, 67, 84, 101, 113, 164–5, 167, 169–70, 174–85, 224
fear 3–4, 6, 8–9, 11, 18, 61, 64–5, 67, 96, 113–14, 127, 129–30, 143, 145, 151, 172–4, 184–5, 204
feelings *see* emotion(s)
feminism 5, 28–9, 198
France 3, 5, 13, 22, 217, 219
  prison policy 85–6, 89–90
FRIEND 19, 153–5
Frigstad, Kirsten 44, 50

Geneva 96–7
Germany 3, 5, 13, 22, 217
  approach to HIV/AIDS 4, 50, 196
  prison policy 87–90
Giuliani, Rudolph 73, 75
gloves 109, 114–17, 149
general practitioners (GPs) 92, 149, 152, 154, 176, 178
grief 130, 154, 184, 192, 204–5, 224, 232
groups
  community 112, 219
  cultural 34, 139
  marginalised 12, 17, 33–4, 42, 46, 66, 82, 110, 124, 129, 131, 194, 222–4
  risk 16, 27, 31–4, 39, 41, 49, 88, 171

support 3, 173, 201
  working 31, 144–5, 183, 196
guidelines 15, 18, 83, 85, 87, 90–1, 97, 100, 110, 114–16, 153
guilt 39, 155, 170, 172–3, 175, 185

haemophilia, people with 3, 5, 20, 31, 39, 67, 144, 198, 230
happiness 201–2
harm reduction 17, 28, 43, 49–50, 90–1, 94, 96–8, 100, 196, 198, 202
health 6, 12, 63, 118, 122, 139, 156, 169, 194, 216, 219
  authorities 5, 41, 44, 141–2, 146, 150
  drug users' 17, 43, 92, 94, 176
  education 13, 145–7, 170, 219, 225
  mental 93, 231
  policy 14, 28, 49, 208
  prisoners' 82, 84, 92, 98, 194
  promotion 18, 147, 156–7, 179
  public 3, 5, 8, 14–15, 17–18, 27–8, 33, 39, 43, 49–50, 61, 72, 77, 83, 89, 91, 97, 100–1, 113, 139–40, 142–3, 145–6, 155, 170, 186, 202, 215–16, 218–19, 221, 225–6, 230
  risks 27, 46, 49
  sexual 111, 143
  sex workers' 17, 40
  visitors 176–8, 183
  women's 164, 173, 175, 198, 222
  workers 17, 19, 45, 49, 119, 139, 145, 152, 167, 172, 174, 178, 193, 232
healthcare 62, 100, 116, 123, 143, 147–8, 157, 178, 219, 221
  prison 82–3, 85, 98–100
helplines 139, 143, 145, 150–1, 153, 155–6

Index

HIV/AIDS
  as chronic disease 4, 7, 110, 230
  crisis 1, 4, 7–9, 14–15, 17–19, 28, 31, 92–3, 110–13, 116–19, 122, 129, 131, 139–42, 149, 154, 164, 168, 170–2, 175, 186, 203–4, 215, 217, 229
  education 13, 16–18, 42, 44–5, 82, 84–5, 88, 91, 94, 100, 139, 142–3, 145–7, 149, 156, 167–9, 171, 217–20, 228
  exhibitions 1, 7–8, 20, 199, 215–16, 219–20, 223–31
  organisations 14, 62, 111, 121, 123, 170, 174, 179–80, 182, 185, 196, 198, 228
  policy 2, 5–6, 12–18, 22, 83–5, 87, 91, 143, 195–6, 229
  see also activism; children; criminalisation; epidemic, HIV/AIDS; hospitals; individual country entries; infection, HIV; pandemic, HIV/AIDS; policy; politics; prison; transmission, HIV; treatment, HIV/AIDS; wards, HIV/AIDS
hospitals 30–1, 37, 62–3, 114, 116, 123, 128–9, 144, 148, 181, 184–5
  HIV/AIDS clinics 173–4, 176–8, 183
  HIV/AIDS wards 18, 110, 117, 125–6
hostility 14, 67, 94, 96, 125, 142–3, 149–51, 153, 157
human immunodeficiency virus (HIV) *see* HIV/AIDS
human rights 6, 46, 167, 198, 201–2, 208
humour 18, 110, 118–19, 129–31

IAS *see* International AIDS Society (IAS)
ignorance 114, 139, 149, 150–1, 157, 201, 209
  'Don't Die of Ignorance' 113, 145, 168, 170
illness 6, 12, 60, 164, 168, 171, 173, 183–4, 219, 225
  AIDS-related 93, 110–11, 114, 117, 120, 126–7, 222
inequality 85, 142–3, 198, 229
  structural 16, 20–1, 143
infection, HIV 3, 6, 28, 68, 151–2, 154–6, 168, 180, 185, 229, 231
  control 114, 127
  modes of 6, 120, 139–40, 144, 151–2, 155–6, 168, 177
  prevention of 40, 170, 186, 217, 228
  rate of 4, 7, 10, 18, 20, 61, 85, 157, 170
  reservoir of 28, 33, 37
  risk of 2, 4, 31, 34, 46, 114, 225, 240
  vectors of 37, 46, 49
information 82, 93, 97, 139, 143, 145, 155, 164, 179, 181, 183, 185, 220, 225
  campaigns 19, 33, 64, 145–6, 153, 156
  lack of 18, 67, 77
  misinformation 143, 180, 184–5, 222, 231
  provision 43–6, 49, 88, 90, 92, 96, 100, 115, 180, 182
  sharing 15, 19
  targeting 33, 88
International AIDS Society (IAS) 20, 215, 217, 225, 228–9
interviews 18, 20, 27, 50, 111–12, 116–18, 126–7, 142, 193, 195–200, 206–9
  see also oral histories
Ireland, Republic of 2, 13, 17, 83–4

approach to HIV/AIDS 91–2, 95–6
prison policy 86, 89–96, 99–100
isolation
  nursing in 109, 114, 116
  in prison 86–7
  social 18, 128, 173, 227, 231
Italy 13
  approach to HIV/AIDS 59–77
  drug use 17, 59, 61, 74–5, 77
  number of HIV/AIDS cases 3, 61, 85, 96
  prison policy 85–6, 88
  see also Casa famiglia

LGBT (lesbian, gay, bisexual, transgender)
  bisexual men 19, 31–2, 34, 154–5
  gay activism 6, 28, 32, 49, 167, 206
  gay men 7, 15–17, 19–20, 33, 59, 118–21, 129–30, 142–3, 151, 154–5, 198, 205, 217, 222, 229
  gay rights 122, 225
  lesbians 117–19, 198, 206
  lesbian activism 28, 32, 49
  lesbian and gay health workers 49, 120, 129
  trans people 118, 198
  see also queer
Liegro, don Luigi di 60, 63, 65–6
London 12, 109, 116–18, 120, 167–8, 182, 205, 222
loss 130, 183, 192, 195, 198, 204–5, 231
Lothian 174, 179–80, 182
lubricant 45–6, 49
Luxembourg 87, 90

Manchester 116, 119–20, 182, 221
marginalisation 4, 12, 15–17, 21, 27, 33–4, 66, 82, 84, 111, 120, 127, 194, 203, 206, 209, 217, 222

masks 109, 114–15
medical
  authorities 66, 72
  change 6, 221, 227, 232
  officers, prison 92, 96–9
  professionals 19, 62–3, 88, 121–3, 140, 144–5, 153, 156, 164, 168, 175, 177–8, 185
  research 13, 62, 122
  response to HIV/AIDS 5–6, 18, 117, 148–9, 186, 222
  services 30, 62–3, 83, 97
  standards 18, 97
medicine
  complementary 219
  construction of boundaries 27
  history of 5, 221, 224, 230
  prison 83, 91
  see also biomedicine
memories 5, 12, 16, 18–19, 110–11, 116, 126, 131, 153, 192–3, 195, 201, 209, 216
men who have sex with men (MSM) 2–3, 34, 140, 202
Middelthon, Anne-Lise 43, 45, 47, 50
migrants 5, 16, 20, 31–2, 194, 224
  see also refugees
Milan 61–62
Ministry of Health, Italian 66, 68–71
misogyny 37, 47, 51
Mitchell, Fiona 178, 180, 183
Mok, Dr Jacqueline 173–4, 176–80, 182, 187, 190–1
  see also Paediatric AIDS Resource Centre
mothers 11–12, 19, 64, 164–86
  see also parents
Mountjoy prison 92–3, 96
MSM *see* men who have sex with men (MSM)
Muñoz, José Esteban 201, 203, 209

Museum of European and Mediterranean Civilizations (MuCEM) 219, 222–3
museum(s) 199, 217–18, 224, 230
   collections 15, 19, 214–16, 218, 224
   role of 20, 214, 216, 218–19, 231
   practices 20, 220–3, 232

narratives 20, 71, 153, 193–4, 197–8, 200, 204–5, 207–8, 216, 222, 224
   disease 171–3
   dominant 39, 195, 216
   historical 4–5, 7, 9, 13, 20, 142, 193
   interpreting 112, 204
National Health Service (NHS) 114, 116, 123, 143
needle
   exchange 90, 93–8, 100, 221, 228
   sharing 43, 61, 85, 98, 139, 168, 177
   see also syringes
Netherlands, the 13, 215, 217, 221, 224, 230
   approach to HIV/AIDS 2, 4, 20, 219, 221–2, 225–6, 228–9
   drug use 94, 221
   number of HIV/AIDS cases 225, 230
   prison policy 85, 89–90, 94
networks 13–14, 143, 166, 173, 193, 207
   international 12, 15, 17, 94, 100, 208
New York 8–10, 13, 59, 73, 75, 174, 207
NHS *see* National Health Service (NHS)
North Wales 149, 151
Northern Ireland 5
   see also United Kingdom (UK)
Norway 2, 12–13
   approach to HIV/AIDS 16–17, 19, 27–8, 31, 33, 44, 46
   attitude to sex workers 16, 27–30, 34, 37, 39–41, 45, 49–50
   drug policy 42–3
   prison policy 86–7
nurses 2, 16, 18, 109–32, 182
   queer 18, 117–20, 129, 131

objects 215, 217–18, 221–2, 224, 230–2
oral histories 1, 8, 16, 18, 21, 27, 83, 110–11, 127, 157, 165, 174, 178, 223
   archiving 192–209
   see also interviews
Oslo 28–30, 32, 34, 40–1, 43, 86

Paediatric AIDS Resource Centre (PARC) 165, 171, 173–4, 178–86
Palermo 74–5
pandemic, HIV/AIDS 1, 3, 6, 20, 201, 215–18, 222–5, 228–31
   see also Covid-19
PARC *see* Paediatric AIDS Resource Centre (PARC)
parents 154, 165, 167, 173, 176–8, 180–1, 183–5, 192
   see also mothers
Parioli, Rome 60, 63, 65–7, 71
partners 19, 31, 33, 40, 117, 154, 167
patients 18, 31, 63–5, 97, 114–29, 132, 140, 148–9, 150–2, 157, 173, 177, 180, 186, 219–21, 226
Penmaenmawr 149–50
picture books *see* books
police 28–9, 40, 44–5, 65, 153, 202
policy
   acquisition 221, 223

drug 6, 42, 73, 194
Dutch HIV/AIDS 229
HIV/AIDS 2, 5–6, 12, 14–15, 17, 27, 167, 193–4, 196–7, 199
Italian HIV/AIDS 17, 73–7
Norwegian HIV/AIDS 16, 28–50
nursing 116, 127
prison 82–101
Welsh HIV/AIDS 18, 143, 149, 157
politicians 28, 44–5, 60, 73, 140, 142, 193, 198
politics 5, 8, 59, 157, 194, 206–8
of HIV/AIDS 5, 46, 49, 207
queer 196, 207
posters 47–8, 88, 170, 218–19, 221, 225, 228
pre-exposure prophylaxis (PrEP) 4, 143, 217, 224, 228
pregnancy 175
prejudice 1, 8, 34, 37, 65, 77, 113, 150
prison 2, 114, 231
activism 84, 89, 95, 100–1
Austria 86
Belgium 86–7, 90
Bulgaria 86, 89
condom provision 84–5, 89, 91
Cyprus 88–9
Denmark 85–6, 90
drug use 17, 73, 85, 90–6, 99, 101
England 83, 86–7, 89
France 85–6, 89–90
Germany 85, 87–90, 98, 196
Greece 86
healthcare 17, 82–3, 85, 91–2, 95, 97–101, 123
HIV testing 85–8, 96, 198
Iceland 89
impact of HIV/AIDS 82–6
injecting equipment provision 85, 90, 95, 97–8, 228

Ireland, Republic of 83–4, 86–7, 89–96, 98–100
Italy 85–6, 88
Luxembourg 87, 90
Netherlands, the 85, 88–90, 94–5
Norway 86–7
officers 17, 84, 92–7, 99
policy 17–18, 82–4, 90–1, 97, 99–100
Portugal 86
prisoners 16, 77, 82, 85–6, 88–9, 92–3, 123, 194, 196, 198
Scotland 85–6, 88, 90
segregation 86–7, 92–3, 96–7, 100–1
Spain 85–6, 88–90
Sweden 86
Switzerland 83–6, 89–91, 96–100
Wales 87, 89
Pro Centre 30, 41, 44–5, 50
prostitution *see* sex workers
Puccini, Fausto Maria 63–5
PWHA (people living with HIV/AIDS) 60, 62, 64, 110–12, 114–16, 119–20, 122–4, 127, 129, 131–2

queer
archival work 195, 200–1, 203, 207
community 110, 117, 154, 167
counter-memory 19, 197, 200, 209
history 195
humour 118
memory 195, 200–1, 209
nurses 18, 110, 117–20, 131
politics 196, 207
spaces 110, 153
theoretical approach 193, 196, 200
understanding of 193, 200, 203–4, 206–7, 209

RCN *see* Royal College of
    Nursing (RCN)
refugees 196, 198
    see also migrants
remembrance 60, 195, 224
resistance 34, 61–2, 203
rights
    drug users' 205
    human 6, 46, 167, 198,
        201–2, 208
    LGBTQ 122, 194, 196, 225
    prisoners' 82, 85, 196, 198
    sex workers' 30, 44, 49–50, 208
    women's 30–1
risk
    factors 33, 67, 95, 156
    groups 16, 27–8, 30–4, 39, 41,
        49, 67, 69, 87–8, 93, 169,
        171, 225
    of infection 2, 4, 13, 31–4, 37,
        43, 45–6, 49, 114, 123,
        125, 154, 174, 225, 230
    perception of 14, 33, 152, 156
    public health 39–40, 74, 86
    reduction 46, 67
Rome 2, 17, 59–62, 66, 72, 77
Royal College of Nursing
    (RCN) 114–15

San Francisco 8–10, 44, 222, 224
Science Museum, London 221–3,
    230
Scotland 18–19, 85–6, 88, 90, 140,
    146, 168–9, 172, 202
    see also United Kingdom (UK)
segregation 125
    prison 83–4, 86–7, 93,
        96, 100–1
    see also isolation
sex
    casual 146, 156
    safe 44–5, 49, 90, 92, 97,
        153–4, 156, 198, 228
    unprotected 70, 85, 169
sex workers 2, 12, 15–17, 27–50,
    77, 169, 194–5, 198, 206,
    222, 225, 228

activism 27–9, 45–6, 50
    as risk group 16, 27, 30–4, 39
    clients of 34, 37, 39–42,
        44–6, 48–9
    criminalisation of 28–9, 50
    diversity of 27, 30, 41
    intersection with drug users
        17, 29–30
    male 41–2
    stigmatisation of 28, 33, 37
sexual
    health 111, 143
    identity 31, 198
    minorities 31, 46, 49
    practices 68, 154
    promiscuity 10, 154, 156
    transmission 6, 31–4, 40, 139,
        143, 198
sexuality 5–6, 32, 92, 111, 127,
    151, 168, 182, 204
social change 6, 31, 34, 50, 112,
    122, 202–3
social workers 14, 16–17, 19,
    28–30, 41, 44–5, 165–7,
    169, 177–9, 182
Spain
    approach to HIV/AIDS 13, 22
    number of HIV/AIDS
        cases 3, 85
    prison policy 86, 88–90
stigmatisation 5–6, 12, 20, 28, 42,
    46, 49, 59–60, 67, 72, 82,
    88, 110, 119, 124–5, 127,
    131, 170–1, 175, 178,
    216, 219, 224, 230
    courtesy 110, 124, 132,
        167, 178
    destigmatisation 34, 44, 46,
        49–50, 82, 180, 222
    self-stigma 37
support 5, 17, 115, 126
    community 6, 94, 117, 142, 157
    family 68
    groups 3, 173
    psychological 114–15
    services 30, 139, 143, 147,
        150, 154

surveillance 31, 125, 176
Swansea 140, 142, 145, 149, 154
Switzerland 2, 85
  approach to HIV/AIDS
    4, 13, 98
  drug use 10–11, 96–7
  prison policy 13, 17, 83–5,
    89–91, 96–100
syringes
  cleaning 42–3, 90
  distribution 42–4, 97–8, 221
  sharing 43, 61, 69–70
  see also needle, exchange

Terrence Higgins Trust (THT) 112,
  123, 147, 151, 156
tolerance 9, 20, 224, 226, 228
training 42, 45, 95, 127, 145,
  165–6, 180, 182
transmission, HIV 4, 6, 77, 154,
  167, 178
  heterosexual 32, 34
  modes of 13, 28, 31–2, 39–40,
    42, 61, 67, 114, 139, 144,
    149, 172
  mother-to-baby 175
  prevention of 68, 98, 143, 169
  in prison 85, 90, 96
  risk of 2, 43, 45
  sexual 6, 31–4, 40, 65, 67, 139,
    157, 198
trauma 40, 153, 155, 175,
  195, 204
treatment, HIV/AIDS 4, 62, 83,
  97, 121–2, 142–3, 148–9,
  156–7, 169, 176–7, 180,
  192, 205, 216, 221
Tyddyn Bach 149–50

unhappiness 193, 201–2
United Kingdom (UK) 2–7, 11, 13,
  18, 59, 146, 167, 179,
  183, 205
  approach to HIV/AIDS 8–9, 11,
    110–32, 142, 145, 168,
    174, 219

  number of HIV/AIDS cases 3,
    110, 117, 140, 144, 168
  prison policy 83, 89, 92, 123
  see also England; Northern
    Ireland; Scotland; Wales
United States of America
  (USA) 2, 59
  approach to HIV/AIDS 3–7,
    31, 114, 129, 144, 194,
    216, 219
  drug use 13, 44, 59, 73

Villa Glori Casa famiglia *see* Casa
  famiglia
volunteers 62, 84, 112, 154–5,
  165, 180

Wales 2, 12–13, 18–19, 87,
  89–90, 139–57
  see also United Kingdom (UK)
wards, HIV/AIDS 63, 86, 109–10,
  112, 117–20, 122–3,
  125–31, 172, 220
WHO *see* World Health
  Organization (WHO)
women 2, 6, 10, 20, 28, 49, 119,
  151–2, 157, 171, 219
  health 164, 198, 222
  HIV-affected 16, 19, 118, 120,
    157, 168–70, 174–5,
    180–1, 186, 230
  prisoners 88, 92, 98
  sex workers 16, 27–32, 34, 37,
    40, 42, 44–6
  see also childbirth; LGBT,
    lesbians; mothers;
    pregnancy
World AIDS Day 3, 67, 139, 146,
  150, 170, 216
World Health Organization
  (WHO) 3–4, 68,
  83–4, 194

Zurich 8, 10, 12, 96–7

EU authorised representative for GPSR:
Easy Access System Europe, Mustamäe tee 50,
10621 Tallinn, Estonia
gpsr.requests@easproject.com

www.ingramcontent.com/pod-product-compliance
Ingram Content Group UK Ltd.
Pitfield, Milton Keynes, MK11 3LW, UK
UKHW021830210426
5322IPUK00004B/119